Bariatric Surgery

*The Best and Worst Decision
I Ever Made*

By
Ed Zenisek

Carra,

Thanks for getting a copy.
I hope you enjoy it!

— Ed Zenisek

ISBN: 1985770296

ISBN-13: 978-1985770294

This book is not intended to be a substitute for the medical advice of a licensed physician. The reader should consult with their doctor on any matters relating to his/her health.

Visit the author's website at http://edzenisek.com/bariatric for more information or to order additional copies.

DEDICATION

To my wife, my love, my rock, for understanding how to deal with my frustration and occasional anger issues and somehow loving me despite it all.

To our family and our friends, without whom my surgery would've sucked way more.

And to our dogs, because they're awesome.

.

Preface

On November 28th, 2017, my wife, Amanda, underwent sleeve gastrectomy. On December 7th, just ten days later, I underwent the same procedure. Those two surgeries were the culmination of almost 20 months of seemingly endless doctor visits, tests, paperwork, and bills.

As my wife and I took our journey into the deep abyss of bariatric surgery, I wondered why nobody told us it would be such a royal pain in the ass. As the pokes and prods turned into frustration, anger, and sticker shock, I decided I needed an outlet. I needed a way to vent my thoughts, other than strangling my doctors or walking into the bariatric center with a shotgun. I know that sounds dramatic, or possibly psychotic, but believe me, I never understood how some post office worker could blow away his co-workers with a machine gun until I tried figuring out how the hell I was going to navigate my bariatric surgery. Now, I understand. I don't condone, mind you, but I understand.

As you may be able to tell by my overly dramatic opening monologue, our experiences weren't always, or even usually, pleasant. Our doctors weren't always great, and I would call our bariatric center office staff mediocre, at best. That said, I will spoil the ending; it was worth it. I don't regret it, not even a little.

There are many other books and media out there that talk about bariatric surgery and use words like "life-affirming," or they might talk about "habits for success." They do a good job of psyching you up for the hard road and lifestyle changes ahead. There's nothing wrong with that. In fact, I think it's wonderful that most books about this subject are positive. It should help you get through the hours of testing, multitude of appointments, and days of waiting for results. Anything you can do to whittle away the hours, while you anxiously hope everything comes back in time for you to make your surgery date, is a good thing. Honestly, I think my book shows a positive outlook on the process in the end. After all, it is a life changing experience that makes people healthier and, ultimately, live longer.

But it isn't easy.

At least it wasn't for us. The entire process took over a year and a half, and every time we thought we crossed the finish line, the doctor's office moved the goal. Having this surgery isn't just about making plans and being ok with changing your lifestyle. It's not just about eating less and cutting carbs. The seemingly endless maze of insurance, Medicare (if applicable), doctor's offices, and doctor's orders make getting the surgery feel more like it's about checking off boxes than about changing your lifestyle.

Keep in mind this is my experience. Every doctor is different, and every patient is too. My wife and I aren't doctors. She's a dispatcher, and I'm a computer programmer... so our opinions don't really mean much in medical circles. Take what I say for what it is, my experience from my point of view. I'm highly confident there are weight loss centers throughout this great land that are bastions of well-planned surgical bliss. Ours was not one of those, at least from our perspective, even though the surgeon turned out to be more than we ever could've hoped for.

In addition to talking about the surgery, I'll also talk about what led us to the decision. Bariatric surgery is a big decision, as any surgeon or nutritionist will tell you, and it took a long time for us to make up our minds to have it done. Amanda and I took the plunge together. Having both of us under the knife within two weeks of each other was quite an experience, and we each had our own issues, pitfalls, and pains. We also each had our own reasons for undertaking the surgery.

Hopefully, if you're considering the surgery, what I've written proves you are not alone... others have been just as confused and frustrated as you are. I hope I can make you laugh about this whole experience, because it's better to laugh than to cry and better to cry than to carry a shotgun into the doctor's office and look menacingly at the receptionist.

Above all, if you're thinking about having bariatric surgery, really thinking about it, then I hope this book helps you make the right decision for you. As I said, I don't regret doing it, and neither does my wife. Or my father. Or my aunt. Or the dozens of people I've met, know, or have otherwise interacted with on our journey. Even though I may be harsh and a bit sarcastic in the book, know that every person I know or have talked to, who has had this surgery, considers it one of the best decisions they've ever made.

Every. Single. One.

As for being the worst decision I ever made, well, that's probably not true. I did sign up for DirecTV once. Also, a book title is all about getting attention. You're reading this, aren't you? The experience was annoying enough to prompt me to write a book, so there's that. There are many words I could use to describe how my wife and I felt about the bariatric and weight loss center where we had our surgery planned, but I think I'll let the experience speak for itself.

In the end, both of us had successful surgeries and went on to significant weight loss. No matter what I write here about the people we interacted with, be they doctors, nurses, staff, or otherwise, I know they were just doing their jobs to the best of their abilities. Many of the experiences I'll share with you are described from the perspective of someone who was either frustrated, angry, disillusioned, or otherwise confused. Looking back, I know I was not always right... or even mostly so.

That said, not only is it more entertaining to write how I actually felt at the time, but it also gives you a window into how you might feel when confronted with the same types of situations, should you do so. Remember, though, there are two sides to every story. This book is my side.

So, now that the niceties are out of the way, we'll begin as most stories do... in the beginning.

I was born on Easter Sunday, 1979...

Chapter 1

The Token Fat Guy

I've always been a big dude. The only time I've ever been small in my entire life was when I was born. I came out screaming and premature in the gas guzzling days of 1979. For the next year or three, I was a happy, healthy, relatively normal baby/toddler, hell bent on doing baby/toddler things. As time marched on, however, the genes from my father's side of the family started to creep into my genetic pool. My father, for as long as I've known him, has been a big dude, too. It wasn't that way when he was young, though. I know that from the pictures. I suppose I could blame my mother's cooking for some of it, but I know better than to blame my mother for anything. In any case, it's easy to blame genetics for being fat. Genetics can't defend itself.

I grew up an only child. My mother gave birth to four children in her life, but somehow, I was the only one blessed enough to survive. Two of my three sisters passed away within hours of being born, and the last passed on after only a day. It happened many years before the doctor slapped my little 3 lb. behind and yelled, "It's a boy, and he is a Keeper!"

So, for all intents and purposes, I grew up as an only child. Even better for me, I was a "mother's miracle," since I was the only child to survive. Mom and Dad rarely denied me anything, so you could say I was a little spoiled. You could also say space is a little big or the ocean is a little wet. I wouldn't call us a rich family by any means, but we certainly ranked as firmly middle class. Living in a modest ranch home outside a small farming community in Illinois, I grew up a country boy. We sat on almost an acre of land, surrounded by corn or beans, depending on the year. The property started as the site of an old school house. Dad saw it as a great opportunity for country living and contracted the house built after I was born.

The property fell on a busy corner, busy for being outside of town, anyway. It was the kind of place that local high school kids used as a landmark. You couldn't miss our Garage. It sat next to the house like a huge brown and white striped monstrosity. Years after I graduated high school, kids I never knew still called the place "Ed's House." I once had a high school junior look at me in awe when she found out I was actually Ed from Ed's House.

As I grew, I continued to get chunkier. My baby fat turned into toddler fat, which turned into kid fat, which turned into… well… just fat. It's sort of vicious, really. When you're a baby, fat is cute! As a toddler, fat is natural, healthy even. When you turn into a kid, fat becomes worrisome, something to talk about in hushed tones. Mothers and fathers proclaim the baby fat is just sticking around for a little longer than other kids, and "he'll thin out eventually." Concerned relatives and friends chatter amongst themselves but refuse to bring it up in polite company. Some parents begin saying phrases like, "Well, he's just big boned," or "He's just a kid; it'll drop off when he starts playing baseball."

I played baseball, and I was still fat.

I wasn't good at it. I was too fat.

Being fat as a kid is a terrible curse. Children are relentless in their teasing, heartless in their insults, and shockingly bad at understanding genetics. Unfortunately, any child different than the status quo falls victim, and I was no different. By third grade, my fatness clearly decided it liked being around, so I became the 'Fat Kid.' I had lots of names, everything from 'Tubby' to 'Eddy Spaghetti in a sack Zen eh zak.' Cruel, but certainly creative.

I remember an occasion in middle school when a kid approached me in the locker room and asked what those marks were on my belly. I had no idea what to say. I thought everyone had those. Another kid, obviously more knowledgeable about such things, mocked, "Those are stretch marks! Pregnant ladies get those!" I felt just as shocked as anyone else in the locker room to discover I bore the marks of a pregnant women on my belly. I was not as amused by it as everyone else seemed to be.

Junior high was tough for me, as I suppose it is for any obese kid.

Ok, for the record, can we all just agree that obese is an awful word? It even sounds fat, like fatness and disappointment, as if the creator of the English language just sighed and rolled his eyes at how fat you've become. Oh. beese. I always hated the word obese. I honestly think the word was at least a little responsible for my desire to have the surgery. At last, I will no longer be obese! Obese Obese. Ugh. Stupid word.

Anyway, looking back, I think junior high was the hardest time for me to be fat in my life. Grade school was bad, and the kids were mean, but they had yet to hone their skills when it came to name calling and ridicule. By junior high, they had verbal torture figured out and were exceedingly efficient at it.

"Hey, lard ass!"

"Dude, just put the Twinkie down, alright?"

"It must've been like giving birth to an elephant. Did your mom survive?"

In a small town, like the one I grew up in, kids end up in school with each other all the way from kindergarten to twelfth grade. Many of the kids I had known since kindergarten suddenly grew a mean streak and felt no remorse whatsoever in fat-shaming me at every opportunity. After all, I presented an easy target. They used me to perfect their bullying skills so that, later, they could mock and tease less obvious targets.

Not all kids were like that, mind you. In fact, most were content to stay out of it. I found that, with a strategy not unlike the turtle, I was able to weather most of the bullying I received. Unfortunately, not all the bullies were content simply using their mouths.

In junior high, we had a gym teacher we all used to call 'Digger.' Someone allegedly caught him picking his nose one day, and it wasn't long before everyone knew. Since this was a school, and we were all immature, the name stuck like an overripe booger. He wasn't a bad guy, not at all, but he was a gym teacher, AKA the mortal enemy of the fat kid.

Gym class, mandatory in Illinois at the time I attended school, became my kryptonite. I hated it. Exercise? Blech. Pullups? Nope, no luck. Run the mile? Right, in 30 minutes maybe. If there's a Dairy Queen at the end.

The only thing I enjoyed about gym was bowling, badminton, square dancing, and that little game where you pop the fuzzy balls in the air with a parachute. Those days excited me, but others terrified me. Physical fitness, weight training, hockey… all those were horrifying to me in different ways, but in all the ways a child could be terrified, nothing terrified me more than wrestling. Remember when I said my strategy for dealing with bullying was not unlike the turtle? That was also my strategy for wrestling. Once a kid had me on my back, my match was over. Fine by me. In fact, I would sometimes intentionally let myself get put down on my back, so I could end the match sooner.

Enter Markus. That's not his real name, by the way. I've changed most of the names in my book to protect the guilty, with a few exceptions for exceptional people. That said, it seemed to me like Markus could bench press a Buick with me in the trunk. Digger figured it would only be fair to match two wrestlers of the same weight class together and decided muscle mass was as good as fat mass. I saw this as a gross miscalculation. Markus saw this as an opportunity to see how much weight he could lift.

The bell dinged. We danced. He grabbed, lifted, and tossed the fat kid as hard as his considerable muscles would allow. I, for my part, flew through the air and landed on my head. My tongue, oblivious to the happenings outside my mouth, rested between my teeth. When I hit the ground, I'm sure it was as shocked as I was.

After I finished spitting bloody bits of tongue meat into the locker room sink, Digger told me to walk it off. I learned an interesting thing about human anatomy that year: The human tongue has amazing regenerative capabilities. I also learned biting off part of your own tongue is a good way to get a parents' note excusing you from wrestling in school… forever.

High school was easier, for me anyway. By the time I made it to high school, most of the bullies I grew up with no longer cared about me. Their 'fat kid' repertoire was all but exhausted, and they moved on to sex and sex-related teasing. Mostly, this focused on kids who may or may not be homosexual. In the 90's, that was a big deal.

Somehow, I found myself almost becoming a mascot of sorts. I became 'Fast Eddy,' and even though the moniker was an obvious play on my size and the irony of calling me fast, I kinda liked it. When I got caught speeding, twice, it only bolstered the nickname. When the second speeding ticket was for going 81 in a 30mph zone, the name became legendary. Ed's House became Fast Eddy's House. I even had many of the same kids, who relentlessly bullied me in junior high, start defending me when some new kid decided to cut his teeth on an easy target. "Hey! Leave him alone. Fast Eddy's cool."

Looking back, I think high school is where my size simply became a part of me. Fast Eddy was a big dude. I would not have been me if I were thin. Even though being big still hurt my popularity and, now that I was a hormone saturated idiot teenager, my romantic options, I contented myself with my fat existence and just accepted it. By then, I allowed insults about my weight to roll off my back easily. I'd heard that stuff all my life. Nobody could say anything I hadn't heard before.

By my junior year, I slotted myself cleanly into the 'token fat guy' role. That's where I felt comfortable. My friends teased me on occasion, but it was the kind of teasing that good friends do to each other. They say something about my weight, I call them stupid, they tell me to go eat a donut… you know, the usual stuff. The rest of the school almost completely forgot I existed. Everyone else had other things on their minds than the fat kid, which was fine by me. I didn't like the spotlight much.

Except when I did.

I enrolled in Drama Club in high school, freshman year, as a matter of fact. I think my interest in drama stemmed from being an only child. Living in the country as an only child meant my best friend was usually myself. My imagination got a lot of exercise. As a result, I loved to ham it up on stage. It's a strange thing about me; I'm a very shy person and don't like being in small groups of strangers very much, but give me a hot microphone and a stage in front of hundreds of people, and I become a completely different person. Drama Club served as an outlet and allowed me to do one of my favorite things... pretend I was someone else. I enjoyed acting in all our high school plays, but none more so than my junior year.

That year, the Drama Club put on a production of *Charly's Aunt* for the community. Because of my sense of humor and because the director's son always got the lead roles, I received the supporting role of Lord Fancourt Babberly. If you're not familiar with Charley's Aunt, it's a play from an older time, when men and women must be chaperoned wherever they go together. The two male leads find themselves hopelessly in love with the two female leads, but alas, they have no chaperone. Fortunately, their aunt Donna Lucia d'Alvadorez is coming to visit and will fill the role nicely. Unfortunately, she is delayed, and the girls are arriving soon. Enter their good friend Lord Fancourt Babberly, who happens to be an amateur theater actor and happens to play an old woman character.

So, in my junior year, I managed to dress up like an old woman and act in front of my entire high school, five o'clock shadow and all. I became Lord Fancourt Babberly, becoming Donna Lucia d'Alvadorez from Brazil (where the nuts come from). Nobody cared that I was fat, and, as a bonus, I even got a peck on the cheek from my high school crush. Of course, it was scripted that way.

Nothing I've ever done in my life earned me as much respect from my peers as that play. Not even close. I can still hear the laughter of the crowd as I fumbled around the stage pretending to be a man playing a woman. Everyone in that theater laughed at me that night, but it was a wonderful, happy, lighthearted laughter that filled my heart with joy. Usually, people laughed at me because I was fat... that night, they laughed because I was funny.

Chapter 2

Someday, I'll Be Thin

You may wonder why I'm telling you all this. After all, what does my childhood have to do with bariatric surgery? I think it's important to understand why I wanted the surgery and maybe why I didn't. Going back that far in my own life helped me to realize how my new life would be different. I encourage you to do the same if you're considering bariatric surgery.

As I've said, I felt comfortable being the token fat guy. Oh sure, I tried over the years to lose weight. Calorie counting, fad diets, eating at Subway. Somehow, deep down, I knew none of those would really work for me. I don't know if it was my genetics or if maybe I didn't even want to lose the weight. Maybe I didn't care enough, or maybe I thought it was too much work to keep in shape. All I can say for sure is this: I never really tried that hard. Any time I did get the gumption to try, the attempt only lasted a few weeks or a couple months, at the most.

Like most folks under the age of 20, I never really felt in danger of health issues. I kept telling myself that, someday, I'll be thin. Someday, I'll lose all the weight and be healthy. I can remember my father trying to lose weight when I was in high school. He traveled over 30 miles to see a nutritionist, who made him write everything he ate in a little book. He could eat only so many starches, so many meats, so many fruits etc. He started talking about how I should go with him because losing weight when you're 17 is so much easier than losing it when you're 47. I had no desire to go. After all, I'd lose the weight someday, but he was my dad, so I rolled my eyes and tagged along.

I tried the little book thing, but I cheated quite a bit. Oh, that massive mound of mashed potatoes? That's a starch. A piece of cake? Dairy, clearly. A half-pound of hamburger smothered with cheese and bacon? One serving of meat. It was easy to cheat, and why deprive myself of the things I love?

Being fat usually means being in love, you know. Being in love with food. My aunt, who had gastric bypass surgery in the late 80's, once told my mom that having the surgery was like losing her best friend.

When the little counting book didn't work for me after a few months, Dad let me drop it. He soldiered on for a little while longer, but, ultimately, it didn't work for him either. Dad knew both of us had a weight issue, and he did what he could for himself. He tried for me too, but I was 17. He was lucky if I did anything he asked me to do at that age, let alone something like going on a diet.

To set the record straight before I go any further, my parents are awesome. I'm extremely fortunate to have them both. Even though I joke about genetics, I do not blame being fat on either of them. Not even a little bit. Everything I like about myself, which is a whole lot, I credit to them.

I said that, so I can say this: they never made me eat my vegetables.

I think having an aversion to vegetables makes losing weight harder than it would be otherwise. People who genuinely like vegetables, like my wife Amanda, have something they can snack on or fill out a meal with that is essentially free, at least when it comes to calories, and dieticians or nutritionists love to see vegetables on your tracking sheet. If you genuinely don't like them, it becomes much harder to find things you can have as a side dish for that all-important 'balanced meal.' Because her parents made her eat her veggies when she was young, Amanda grew accustomed to them, in some cases, even fond of them.

I hate vegetables. Always have. I once read an article on the internet about hating vegetables, where one of the comments said something like, "Anyone who says they don't like vegetables is stupid. That just means they haven't tried hard enough. There are so many ways to make them! If you don't like them, then you just haven't found the right way to make them."

For some reason, that comment stung, even if it did come from some nameless shmoe on the internet. It's like that person was saying I'm too much of an idiot to figure out a way to make yard waste taste like mana from heaven. Oh, if only I were smart enough to find the magic spice that could turn a brussel sprout into a Ho Ho or turn some asparagus into pixie sticks. Seriously though, if I could do that, I wouldn't be a programmer. Iron Chef, here I come!

I've tried vegetables of all kinds, cooked all kinds of different ways. I've found them to range from palatable to gross to downright gag-inducing. Nothing I've tried has been what I would consider delicious, with the possible exception of a salad. So long as it has the proper dressing. And croutons. And some meat. And a bun.

I think my disdain for vegetables is one reason dieting doesn't work much for me. What I should say instead is it's one reason I can't stick to a diet. Of course, dieting works... it's not the diet that's at fault. It's the person straying off the diet because a handful of broccoli and some celery sticks just doesn't do it for them.

You might notice I'm blaming everything but myself for my size. I'm not stupid though; I know it's not all about genetics, or not liking vegetables, or even being Fast Eddy. The truth is, I like food. A lot. When I have access to it, I eat it. I like to make excuses, but nobody puts the food in my mouth for me, and nobody plops my fat butt on the couch for me either.

Any nutritionist worth anything will tell you the key to losing weight is diet and exercise. Even the phrase has become a cliché. It's true though, unfortunately. I got fat at a young age because I ate too much of the wrong things and played video games more often than I went outside. Hell, I still do. That stuff is fun though, and food is good. You can't just stop eating it either. If you have an alcohol addiction, you can safely never have another alcoholic drink in your life. Not that I'm trying to make alcoholism sound like a walk in the park, but people who are fat need to eat. Everyone needs to eat. If you don't eat, you die. Makes going cold turkey kind of hard. Could you imagine if an alcoholic had to have a beer at least once every couple of days?

I think a lot of folks who have never struggled with weight just don't understand how hard it can be. I don't pretend to understand how hard it is for an alcoholic, how could I? I don't have that problem. I'm lucky that way. When I say that, I'm not trying to mock… I really do feel like I'm a very lucky person regarding addiction. I used to smoke about a half-pack a day. When I decided I wanted to quit, I just quit. Just like that. One day, I woke up and said, "This is expensive. I don't think I want to smoke anymore."

Food though, food is different. I liked smoking. I love food. I wish there was an easy way to quit food sometimes. I'd settle for a patch, like a nicotine patch, only maybe it smells like pie. As long as it doesn't smell like brussel sprouts. Blech.

Once, driving to a college class, I heard an ad on a wacky morning radio show about this fat burning pill that would send your metabolism into overdrive and help you burn calories sitting still, no vegetables required. The guy in the ad said he'd lost a bunch of weight and still got to eat whatever he wanted. Sounds like a winner! Two weeks later, I had two bottles of the little pills and couldn't wait for the fat to melt off.

What actually happened were terrible shakes, nausea, cold sweats, and a version of butt chunder that I've not experienced before or since. No wonder the dude lost weight.

And, of course, who hasn't tried the Subway diet? Slap some veggies on a bun with some meat and they become like the backup singers in a band… even if they're not great, they contribute to the greatness of the whole. One summer, I was bound and determined to lose weight after I caught myself needing two foot-long sandwiches to feel full. I was shocked that I felt like I needed that much, so I found some willpower for a change. I cut my typical two foot-long sub meal down to a single six-inch sub with no mayo or chips and started jogging on a treadmill almost every day. Guess what? It worked! I began to lose weight. Once I was down about twenty pounds, I felt like I'd accomplished something, so I needed a reward. My reward, as you can probably guess, was not good for me. I took a few days off. Then I took a few more. Pretty soon, the weight was starting to creep back up, but I thought, "Eh, it's ok. I'm nowhere near where I was. I'm still doing good." Fast forward a couple of months, and I was right back where I'd started.

As I said, I don't think I wanted to lose the weight. Not really. Psychologically, I'd accepted my size as part of who I was, and so had my friends. I wouldn't be the same Fast Eddy if I lost a bunch of weight. Not that my friends would ever discourage me from losing it, but I don't think they saw it as a problem. Neither did I, to be honest. After all, if it did become a problem, it was one for future Fast Eddy to solve. I'd be thin someday. As for now, it wasn't a big deal. I was young and strong, with no need for ongoing medication or regular doctor visits.

That began to change around the time I started going to college. It took me a couple years to figure out I wanted to be a programmer, so I didn't start college until the age of 20. Weight related things, other than just being winded going up stairs or not being able to run a mile, began to creep into my daily life. At first, it was simple; my blood pressure would be a bit higher than normal during a routine checkup, or sores would crop up every now and then between my thighs or around where the top of my pants would rub my skin. Stuff that doesn't really set off too many alarm bells when you're young.

Being completely unable to walk one morning became my first sign of impending doom. My right foot felt swollen, and I couldn't put any pressure on it. A trip to the doctor revealed the cause to be gout. Called the "rich man's disease," gout tends to afflict those with a sedentary lifestyle more so than active folks. After a few days, the pain dissipated, and I found myself able to walk again. About a year later, the gout came back with a vengeance. The doctor that time put me on a medication to control it, and when I asked how long I needed to take the pills, he said, "Forever."

That was a rough revelation for me. Suddenly, I was mortal. Suddenly, I had something I must take to stay healthy and prevent myself from excruciating pain. I had to take it every night! Oh, the humanity! For the rest of my life, I would be dependent on a medication.

It was such a shock that I immediately went into the first stage of grief: Denial. Well, I rationalized, I'm still young. It's not like I really need this medication. Doctors are always prescribing things people don't really need. I'm not even sure it's gout. It's probably just a sprain or something. Stupid doctor! There's the second stage: Anger.

I even looked up the drug, Allopurinol, on the web. This was a mistake. The side effects are horrifying. Words like *toxic epidermal necrolysis* and *interstitial nephritis* scream off the page in bright blue hypertext. Clicking on them is not recommended, but I clicked anyway. The imagery kept me up at night. I decided that no amount of gout pain could compare to the terrors I found within the side effect list on the internet. That's another stage: Bargaining.

In 2003, I began working as a Slot Technician at a Casino in Illinois, and that meant walking the casino floor all night every night. My weight stabilized, and the gout symptoms didn't come back. In 2007, I followed my parents to New Mexico, where they retired. I lucked out and found a job as a web developer at New Mexico State University. I had a desk job, and my waistline began to tell the story. After about three years there, I had the worst gout attack of my life. We're talking rolling around the house in a computer chair with only my underwear on kind of bad. Even putting on pants or letting a sheet from my bed rest on my foot resulted in the kind of agony for which screaming into a pillow was the only respite. Depression? Check off that stage of grief.

After that, I began taking my Allopurinol every day. I still do. I haven't had an attack since, and I think taking one pill a day every day for the rest of my life is a small price to pay. That's acceptance.

I look back on that time now and chuckle a little. I was naïve. The number of pills I swallow daily today makes that one pill seem like a single flower in a bouquet of roses, if roses had terrible side effects and made your poo look funny. I've added blood pressure medication, a daily multi-vitamin, and a water pill to my regimen. Unfortunately, I've also added metformin and sitagliptin. If you've never heard of either of those drugs, then congratulations... you're not diabetic. I come from a not-so-proud family tradition of diabetes. My grandmother had it, my father has it, and now I have it. I think, if I had to give you any reason for having bariatric surgery, controlling my diabetes would be the answer. It's incredible how closely related your weight, your diet, and diabetes becomes in your overall health. Diabetes is a monster that preys on you your entire life unless you can control it.

Chapter 3

The Evil of Diabetes

Diabetes is insidious.

It creeps up on you like a stalker, robbing your body of its ability to handle sugar. Normally, your pancreas makes enough insulin to deal with whatever sugar you take in, but when diabetes shows up, it makes your body gradually get worse at using the insulin your pancreas creates. This causes your glucose (sugar) levels to rise, which begins wreaking havoc on your body in all kinds of ways.

I remember my paternal grandmother when I was very young. Unfortunately, she died when I was twelve. Margaret Zenisek was a wonderful grandma, always fawning over her grandchildren. She liked to call herself the 'kissing bandit' because, whenever she first saw us, she would run over and slather us with kisses. They weren't the sloppy, wet, nasty crazy aunt kind but the sweet, loving, beautiful grandma kind. She was amazing, and that's how I like to remember her.

Diabetes didn't take her directly, but it was there, responsible, lurking in the shadows while she wasted away at the relatively young age of 64. I remember bits and pieces of how the disease affected her. I was still young and care-free, so the concerns of old age were other peoples' concerns. Every now and then, though, I would get a flash of how the disease affected her life.

Diabetes is insidious.

It's also slow and sneaky. It happens so slowly that you don't even notice, especially when you're young. When you get older, you start going to the doctor once or twice a year. When you're young, you may not go for years at a time. The only way to diagnose diabetes is with a blood test. By the time your diabetes is bad enough for you to have symptoms, it's already doing serious damage to your body. If you're overweight, even if you're young, you should at least get a glucose meter and check your glucose levels every now and then, just to be sure.

Type 2 diabetes, like many diseases, has differing levels of severity. Type 1 diabetes is an altogether different monster, which, thankfully, I know little about. Type 2 starts out mildly enough. You go to the doctor, he says something along the lines of, "Your A1C came back a little high on that last blood test. It's 6.1, and we'd like to see it below around 5.8. This may be a sign of prediabetes."

"Ok," you think. "Prediabetes. That's not real diabetes. That's like, totally ok. I don't have it. I may get it someday, but there's still time to fix it, right?"

Yes, there is time to fix it. I didn't. Neither did my dad or my grandmother. Or my best friend. It's hard. It's the life-changing, diet and exercise, making a commitment to your health kind of hard. People who are overweight or obese (ugh) don't tend to like doing that kind of stuff, so they don't tend to fix it.

If you don't fix it, like me, then on your next visit your doctor will say something like, "Ok, so your A1C came back at 6.4 this time. That's still high. Since you have two tests in a row that came back that high, you officially have prediabetes. I'm going to prescribe 250mg of metformin twice a day, so we can get this under control."

Oh no, another one of those forever medications.

Believe it or not, at this point there is still time to fix it. The real key is cutting out sugar from your diet. That's not as easy as it sounds though because like I said before, diabetes is insidious.

Sugar seems like a straightforward thing to cut from your diet. Stop eating Ho Ho's and Ding Dongs. Done. Not so fast. Sugar is the primary energy source for your body, and I'm sure that folks like Michael Phelps and Ernie Banks didn't get their athletic ability from Ding Dongs. Sugar isn't just the sweet stuff they put in delicious treats and candy bars... sugar is everywhere. Every. Where.

A whole lot of food, good food, is made up of stuff they call carbohydrates. If you don't know what a carbohydrate is, it's basically anything that tastes good that isn't meat. Carbohydrates, or carbs, are found in almost all food, but especially starchy stuff like bread, pasta, beans, or rice. I'm no nutritionist, and I have no idea how this all really works, but if you look on a food label you can see it. Carbs are broken down into sugar (simple carbohydrates), and fiber (complex carbohydrates).

For your body, anything that is a carbohydrate and isn't a fiber is sugar, even if it isn't listed as sugar itself on the label. By the time your body gets done with it, it all turns into glucose. Glucose is the thing that diabetics care about the most because it dictates their blood sugar level and their A1C (which is a long-term blood sugar measurement). Those measurements tell you how well controlled your diabetes is. The higher your average blood glucose level, the more health issues you start to face. Up to and including death, of course.

If you go to your doctor and have an A1C higher than 6.5 then it's likely they will diagnose you with full blown type 2 diabetes. It's at this point that you're considered diabetic and may, or may not, start panicking about it. It's likely your metformin dose will be upped to 1000mg twice a day and, if you continue to show high A1C levels, you might get another drug like sitagliptin or glipizide or any other of a dozen different drugs with all kinds of interesting names. This is all to prevent you from needing the end all be all of diabetes medications: insulin injections.

At this point, if you don't deal with it, you're almost certainly going to need insulin. Diabetes is insidious. It makes the insulin your body makes less and less effective, and, eventually, you make less and less of it. Insulin is responsible for dealing with glucose in the blood. I'm not going to pretend like I know how this works, but, over time, a high level of blood glucose can cause things like eyesight damage, nerve damage, and even necessitate the amputation of limbs. Nasty stuff, to be sure.

Once your body no longer creates enough insulin on its own to deal with the sugar you intake, you need to start adding insulin on your own to keep your glucose at a safe level. The problem with this is that insulin is a very powerful hormone, and sugar is actually very necessary for you to have in your body.

Low levels of blood sugar can cause things like blurry vision, fatigue, and headache if the levels are beginning to get low. If they get very low you can faint, have a seizure, or even slip into a coma. It's even called a diabetic coma if this happens because a diabetic took too much insulin for their glucose level. That's the hard part. If you start adding insulin to your body, then you are now personally responsible for making sure you add the right amount. Up to this point in your life, your pancreas did that for you. It knows what it's doing. "Hey, live your life," says your pancreas, "I got this." With advanced type 2 diabetes though, your pancreas is screaming, "Help me dammit! What have you done? Why is this not working?" Now it's your job, and most folks aren't as good at it as their pancreas used to be.

If you get to the point where you inject insulin, your life changes pretty much right away. You live and die by the glucose meter. Three, four, or even more times a day you must prick your finger and bleed into a little strip while you wait for a machine to beep at you and reveal your magic number. If your number is high, say 175, then you need to add some insulin. If your number is low, like 78, then you definitely do not. The amount of insulin you take is proportionate to the number you get when you take your test. You are responsible for getting it right. Get it wrong and you could fall into a coma. Scary stuff.

My grandmother got it wrong at least once while I was around. I don't think that she was very good at keeping track of her glucose levels, but I was a kid and really had no idea what was going on. All I remember is that we were shopping at a store somewhere and Grandma wasn't feeling good. She started to act very sleepy, and Dad started to seem a little worried. The sleepier Grandma got, the more worried Dad got. Eventually, someone from the store brought Grandma a wheelchair and when she fell into it, Dad hollered at my mom to go get some juice. Mom ran to wherever that store kept the orange juice, and they didn't even pay for it. They just ripped the container open and poured it into Grandma's mouth.

She ended up being ok – that day. Eventually, it got her in the end, though. Like I said, diabetes wasn't directly responsible, but if she didn't have it, there's not a doubt in my mind she would've lived a much longer, happier life.

Diabetes scared my dad. He saw what it did to Grandma and knew the repercussions. I've said my father was always a big guy, at least for as long as I've known him. With it running in the family like it does, him becoming a diabetic was almost an inevitability.

He cried when he got the diagnosis. It scared him so badly that he vowed to control it. He was going to beat it, make sure he ate right, and did everything he could to keep the disease at bay. Eating right wasn't really that hard in my house. Mom and Dad both were good cooks, and they made food that was good for us almost every night. There was the occasional fried chicken, pizza, or take out hamburger, but these were the exceptions, rather than the rule. In the end, though, he still had to inject insulin to manage his diabetes.

He did an amazing job. His injections were meticulous all the time. I can't remember a single time in my life when my father needed to eat a sugar pill or drink orange juice because he mis-dosed his insulin. I'm not sure he ever even felt woozy. My memories of him in this stage of his life always include a carrying case for his insulin and his glucose meter. If a son can be proud of his dad, then I'm proud of him for controlling diabetes so well with insulin.

I think that may not have been good for me, though, in the long run. Don't get me wrong. I have nothing but admiration for the way he handled the disease. All I'm saying is that he never scared me the way my grandmother scared him. He handled it so well that I never felt like it was an issue. When I finally got my diagnosis, I just brushed it off. I knew it was coming. Grandma had it, Dad has it, so I'll have it too... someday. When that day came, it didn't seem like a big deal to me, much less a surprise.

I was bummed, of course, but not terribly. I received all the pamphlets, all the warnings, got scheduled to go see a self-help group. I even got a little diabetic cookbook. When I got home, it all went in the trash. I still had time to fix it. I would. Plenty of time. I'll stop eating chocolate. No more ice cream. Well, maybe a little, but just a little.

Diabetes is insidious, and it's persistent and progressive. I changed nothing about my lifestyle, so diabetes just kept steaming along. Pretty soon, I was at the max dosage of metformin and staring to take Januvia (sitagliptin). I think it was the Januvia that finally started me thinking about the surgery more seriously. That shit's expensive. When my doctor finally gave me an ultimatum and said, "The next time you see me and your A1C is over 7, we're going to need to start you on insulin." That's when it hit home that I needed to do something real, and bariatric surgery may be something I really need, rather than a passing thought. When I looked up the cost of insulin, the reality hit me in the head like a sack of stevia.

Take my health from me? Meh, no biggie. Take my money? Now, I'm ready to fight.

Chapter 4

Married Without Children

I met my wife Amanda for the first time in November of 2011. We found each other at an online dating site because I'm shy and terrible at talking to women. She was there for the quizzes. We hit it off well, and we seemed to have a lot in common. I used to be a Boy Scout, she a Girl Scout. We both drove Ford trucks. Family is paramount to each of us, and we're both very close to our respective parents. Now, we're very close to each other's parents, too.

Another thing we had in common was being overweight. We both knew the struggle of dealing with food and diets and both knew how it felt to be the butt of jokes and subject of ridicule. Both of us were shy with the opposite sex, which I'm sure had to do with our appearance. Amanda is a beautiful woman, but at the time we met, she was overweight enough to cause most men to pass. As a large person myself, I felt some comfort in that.

It may sound strange, but there's something about approaching a thin girl as a fat guy, and I'm sure the other way around, that makes it almost feel like a taboo. Being fat, I was conditioned to thinking I was also repulsive to most women. With Amanda, I didn't feel that way. Part of it was her size, but a lot of it was her attitude. She didn't care how big I was.

If my waistline was a result of not liking vegetables much (among other things), hers was a result of becoming a dispatcher for the Sherriff's Office after high school. While she was in school, she kept active enough to stay at a manageable weight. I don't think anyone would've called her thin, but fat was probably a stretch. She's a tall girl and solidly built. No matter how much weight she loses, she'll never be what folks would consider 'thin.' Once she found a sedentary job, however, the lack of activity and the addition of a dispatcher diet made keeping her weight under control very hard.

Genetics also play a role in Amanda's weight. Her mother fights tooth and nail to keep herself from being overweight. She keeps herself on crazy diets with less than 1000 calories a day and walks miles and miles each morning to burn off what little she eats. It works for her though; she keeps the weight off. For some reason, Amanda's mom seems like a gladiator wrestling a tiger all the time. Sometimes, the tiger gets a bite or a paw on her, but mostly, she fights it back. She never wins completely though, so she's always fighting it. I'm sure a whole lot of folks could relate to that.

I'm sure the fact that she is the most excellent baker ever to grace this side of heaven doesn't help. Kim, Amanda's mom, should have a song written about her, called "Devil went down to New Mexico and Got His Ass Kicked in a Baking Contest." She actually made the cake for our wedding and, to this day, it's the best cake I've ever eaten.

Kim is the type of person who bakes a phenomenal cake and then won't eat more than a small slice because it's too many calories. Amanda and I, unfortunately, don't have that kind of self-control. It's interesting to me how many times I hear people talk about their mothers or grandmothers doting over them and telling them to watch their weight or get healthier, while making a huge pot of some artery clogging, coma inducing, carb saturated recipe passed down by the angels themselves. They then, somehow, expect folks to eat that amazing bowl of heart attack special and stay healthy at the same time. Kim is that way but without the pressure. She doesn't ask you to try her baking or make you take desserts home with you when the party's over. But you do. Of course, you do. When you hear choir music every time you take a bite, you just can't say no, ya' know?

I'm not sure if I should say fortunately or unfortunately here, but either way, Amanda inherited some of Kim's baking prowess, as well. I remember the first birthday I had after we started dating. She made me this chocolate coconut cheesecake that seemed barely to fit on my kitchen counter. I'm a sucker for cheesecake, and I don't remember exactly how she found that out, but she did. Damn, that was some good cheesecake, and it was all mine. I shared some with her on my birthday when she brought it over, but we weren't living together yet, and she went home that night. Since we lived an hour away from each other while we dated, we didn't usually see each other until the weekend. That meant I had a week to lay into that cake all by my lonesome.

By the time I asked her to marry me, any semblance of weight control I might've had since my days as a slot technician was long gone. Between the bachelor life, Kim's cooking, Amanda's cooking, and genetics, of course, it seems my waistline didn't stand a chance.

We married on September 21st, 2013. The cake might've had something to do with it, but mostly, it was the girl. I've never had a woman in my life treat me as well as Amanda did and still does. We make an amazing team, and I feel like we could do almost anything if we put our minds to it.

Almost anything.

As soon as we were married, we decided we wanted a family. We started trying pretty much right away. Amanda always said she wanted three children, but being an only child, I think I'd be ok with any number higher than one. Only children are crazy. And spoiled.

We tried and tried. It was fun, sure, but after a while, it began to seem like maybe it just wasn't going to happen. Pretty soon, folks around us started having babies. We were at that age when all our friends were getting married, having kids, and starting their families. We wanted that too, and it's a strange feeling being both excited for and jealous of another expectant mother.

We gave it a year. We read online that you should give it the old college try for about that long before you contact a doctor. Once the year was up, we found a reproductive specialist and began regular trips to the doctor's office. The first step, of course, was to determine if each of us could even have a child.

My job in that regard was to drop some kids off at the clinic and see if they could swim. They could. According to the doctor, they were regular little Olympic gold medalists. Yay me.

That meant it was likely Amanda that was having the issue, and that turned out to be the case. They diagnosed Amanda with PCOS. Polycystic ovary syndrome is not uncommon, about 2-20% of child bearing age women, depending on how you define the diagnosis. It is also one of the leading causes of infertility among women. Weight is a contributing factor and affects how severe the disease becomes.

Once we learned it was almost certainly PCOS causing the fertility issue, we were both saddened and relieved. Saddened because my wife was diagnosed with an incurable disease but relieved it didn't necessarily mean she could not have children. PCOS makes it more difficult and increases the likelihood that fertilization will not take place during any given cycle, but it does not mean it can't happen.

The next step was regular monthly treatments. It was time to break out the calendar because, baby, we're on a schedule now. You ever see a sitcom where the guy and the girl are trying to get pregnant? The guy is with his buddies and glances at his watch, "Whoops! Time to go." He runs out the door and into his wife's loving embrace, where bow chicka wow happens and life is good. It's almost just like that. Except that, instead of a watch, it's a calendar, and instead of a bow chicka wow, it's like a bow chicka wow here we go again, even if you're not in the mood. While you're on fertilization treatments, it's very important to be on schedule. I remember several times when my wife and I had the uncomfortable realization that we would be staying with relatives when the day came. Bow chicka hush hush.

After a few months of that with no success, it was time to up the ante. We moved on to intrauterine insemination, and it's every bit as cold and dull as it sounds. The most exciting part about it was being even more of a slave to the calendar.

A certain number of days after a period, she had to take this certain drug, and then a certain number of days later, she had to go to the pharmacy and get a certain shot, bring it to the doctor's office, and have it administered. Then the next day, I had to go in and drop some more kids off at the clinic, so the following day she could go in and 'pick them up,' which means having them more or less injected with something not unlike a turkey baster.

The shot was a couple of hundred dollars a pop, and the other medications, including pregnancy tests, weren't cheap either. The visits add up, and soon, you're making the equivalent of a new car payment each month for the outside chance that maybe, just maybe, you can be blessed with something that a couple of randy teenagers can create in the back seat of their father's Coupe Deville without even trying. Their first. Damn. Time.

But I'm not bitter.

After about six months we had to stop. Not only was the expense becoming prohibitive for us, but Amanda had to stop the medications anyway. You can only safely take them for so long before you need a break. Let me also set the record straight here for anyone thinking I'm a cheapskate: I would give anything I own to be able to conceive a child with my wife. We weren't paying for a child; we were paying for a chance. Each time we did, it felt like the chances got slimmer and slimmer.

It takes a mental toll, as well. Every time my wife felt queasy, was it morning sickness? Oh, she has a strange craving, maybe she's pregnant! Every time she kept a secret from me for a surprise of some kind, I fretted and worried that it might be a child, or it might not. It honestly began to affect my mood. Valentine's day, my birthday, any holiday became a minefield of wondering if that would be the day she told me. She never got the chance.

Throughout it all, one thing kept coming up. Each time we saw the fertility specialist, she told Amanda the best way to reduce the infertility of PCOS was to lose weight. Women who lose a significant amount of weight often become very fertile, the doctor would say. It's either that or in-vitro, and if I thought a car payment was expensive, in-vitro meant taking out a second mortgage.

We had a lot to think about.

Chapter 5

Dad, the Trailblazer

My father had bariatric surgery in late 2015. It took many years, a few different insurance companies, and different doctors to fulfill his dream of surgery. My parents retired to New Mexico in 2005, and Dad had been trying for years even before they moved. Nothing ever seemed to line up. Either insurance wouldn't cover him or the requirements to get it done were just too much to bear. When he first started trying, in the 90's, many insurance companies didn't cover the procedure because it was, and still is, considered 'elective'. That means it's not medically necessary, so it gives insurance companies a way out of covering it. My father even had his primary care physician draft a letter to the insurance companies, telling them, in my father's case, it was medically necessary to facilitate a standard quality of life.

They didn't care. It was a procedure they didn't have to cover, so they didn't cover it.

Fast forward to around 2012 and my father was really beginning to show the effects of his obesity. By that time, he was in his late 60's, and his joints were starting to bear the brunt of his weight problem. He couldn't stand for very long, and for the first time in my life, he stopped working on all but the simplest projects around the house because they were too painful. I can remember noticing how, whenever he entered a room, the first thing he looked for was a place to sit down. If he couldn't find one, he looked for a way to get out and find a place to sit down. I got used to looking for places to sit when I was with him and making sure he would have a place if he needed it. Good public seating became a favorable feature of our family outings, and we stopped frequenting places that didn't have it.

In 2015, Dad saw an advertisement for a local Bariatric Surgeon. It reinvigorated his desire for the surgery, but he'd been met with so many roadblocks before, he was a little hesitant to go forward with it. I think the thought of his own future was what put him over the edge, though. He realized he couldn't get a handle on his weight problem by himself, and if he wanted to see grandchildren someday, he needed to extend his life. It seemed surgery was the best way to do that.

So, he made an appointment.

It was a long road. He ended up going to the same bariatric and weight loss center that Amanda and I would go to years later, but he had a different surgeon. For some reason, the office there was incredibly inefficient in handling all three of our surgeries. I will sing high praises for the two surgeons who did our three procedures and the nurses who attended, but the office was a hot mess the whole time. It made jumping through the necessary hoops quite frustrating. Like trying to herd cats. On fire. With a water hose.

When the time finally came, he chose the sleeve gastrectomy. It's been very successful. Originally, he wanted to have the lap band because it seemed less invasive and a little less permanent. He changed his mind after going to a few bariatric support group meetings and hearing from other folks who had surgery of varying types. He found out the sleeve is a far more successful procedure than the lap band. Success, in this case, is measured by the number of people who have the procedure done and can say, after several years, they've met and maintained their target weight.

I've examined the studies, and if you believe the statistics, it's true that the lap band success rate is a little disappointing. I'll talk more about the different types of bariatric surgery and what I think of them a little later, but for now, I'll just say I think Dad made the right choice. He does too. Before he went into surgery, he weighed almost 330 lbs. Last I talked to him, last week, he was down to 225. He's had ups and downs since the surgery, but I'd say he's done very well.

My father's weakness is candy and sweets. Even now, after the surgery, if we have candy laying around in a bowl in the house, he always grabs a handful. He can pass up bread, fried foods, and stuff like pizza without a problem, but if there's a slice of cake or a piece of pecan pie around, he just can't say no. I guess it runs in the family.

Post-op, of course, the pieces of pie or cake he eats are very small. He just gets a taste, and it seems to please him enough that he's satisfied. I always envied him for that after his surgery. Oh, to be satisfied by a thin wedge of cake, instead of needing the cake equivalent of a side of beef.

On the Fourth of July, the year after Dad's surgery, we attended my sister-in-law Nicole's birthday party. Nicole's birthday is on July 4th, so we always end up having a birthday/Independence Day party. That means lots of fireworks and lots and lots of sweets. Since she's my sister-in-law, her mother is my wife's mother, and Kim (whom I talked about before - remember the devil getting his ass kicked?) does most of the baking. Dad was powerless against that level of baking mastery.

About eight months post-op, Dad could pretty much eat whatever he wanted in small portions. He ate his dinner, little bits of everything, and then couldn't help but help himself to dessert. Besides the stuff Kim baked, other partygoers had also procured some sweet treats for the birthday girl. Dad decided to try a little bit of them all. Remember, sweets are his weakness, and it's easy to rationalize just a small bite of this and a small bite of that. They're all small bites, so what?

The so what came after the party. Once it began to get dark, we all drove to a local therapy center, where Nicole worked. They had a nice get together set up in the parking lot for employees, and it provided a perfect view of the fireworks. Everyone going to the event was kind enough to bring food, and it was almost all sweet stuff. Dad was starry-eyed. Once again, the temptation proved too much to resist, and very small portions of a whole lot of sweets found their way into my dad's extra small-sized stomach. Soon, it was time to view the fireworks. This was in Alamogordo, New Mexico, and the fireworks were beautifully framed by the Sacramento Mountains. It was a gorgeous display, and I'll never forget the booming echo of the reports as they rolled through the valleys of the mountains. In the middle of the show, I looked over at my father. What I saw was both distressing and amusing.

Dad was sitting there with the look of a man who had eaten a cow, hooves and all. With sweat rolling down his face and a pained expression, he looked at me and said, "Son, you may be in the state of New Mexico, but I'm in the state of misery."

I think that was the worst time he had post-op. You hear stories about folks eating too much and throwing up or even getting dumping syndrome, but Dad never had any of that. I know I make it sound like he's a regular vacuum when it comes to sweet stuff, but the reality is much milder. When that stuff is available, sure, he partakes, but my parents do a good job of keeping sweet stuff out of the house. After all, he has lost over 100 lbs. Either he's keeping to his regimen, or cake in my parent's house has magical properties. I can attest it is not the latter.

Dad was lucky in that he already had a lot of the post-op diet behaviors built into his daily routine. The meals he ate were good balanced meals. He just ate too much. As I said, he had a weakness for sweets, which compounded the issue and is still a problem, but without the large stomach giving the orders anymore, it's not as hard to resist. One of the biggest things my dad had going for him was that he likes leftovers.

Oh boy, does he. My father is the kind of guy that will cook a humongous pot of soup on Sunday and eat it for lunch and dinner every day for weeks until its gone. If it's a food he likes, he never gets tired of it, and he doesn't care if its leftover or not. He'll order a huge amount of food at a restaurant, fully understanding he won't even touch most of it until later in the week, when he reheats it in a microwave somewhere. He loves to order a full rack of ribs from a local steak place and then grin as the servers gawk while he puts the entire thing into a to-go container, having only eaten the side of chili and vegetables that came with the meal. He'll then brag to anyone who will listen how he'll get four meals out of that at home.

Dad is at the point now, where he can eat anything he wants. He'll even have pizza, pasta, or a roll, on occasion. It's a rare thing for him to have a carb-laden meal, but it does happen, and it allows him to feel like he's not being robbed of some of the foods he enjoys. It's like a special treat for him, and he's usually aware of his diet enough to know where he is with his protein, carb, and calorie intake to keep things at the right place.

He is human, though, and it wasn't too long ago that his weight began to creep back up to where he became uncomfortable with it. He got just a little complacent and quit monitoring his intake. Once he hit that point, he took control of his eating habits again, made easier by having the surgery, and his weight began to drop almost immediately. One thing the doctors and the internet keep telling us is that this surgery is a 'tool.' It's something to help you lose weight, but it won't do it for you. Seems to me it's an incredibly powerful tool, like the jaws of life or an aircraft carrier. As soon as he'd made up his mind again to lose the weight, it came off. He had to eat right and keep his calorie count down to where it needed to be, but it wasn't agonizing. He didn't feel deprived or hungry; he just… changed the way he ate a bit.

I think that's one thing I looked forward to the most as a result of my own surgery. That big powerful tool. The ability to make up my mind to lose the weight and just do it by eating right and having the occasional treat. Before the surgery, doing that same thing would cause me to hover around 280 lbs. because the portions were so big. I felt like they had to be to satisfy me. But oh, to be able to eat a small meal and feel full! The ability to eat just a little and feel satisfied! What a wonderful thought.

My father constitutes just one of the many success stories I've heard from countless people who have had or have known someone who had weight loss surgery. I've not heard a single bad experience, overall, from anyone I know. My father is also an inspiration to me and has been my entire life.

While his weight may not have been a great example to set, I consider every other facet of who he is to be something I aspire to be. Once he got his weight under control, I figured it would be only a matter of time before I felt compelled to do the same.

Chapter 6

Do as I Say, Not as I Do

Before I begin talking about the actual journey my wife and I took to our bariatric surgery, I want to say something plain and simple. What I've written in this book is my opinion and nobody else's. I am not a doctor, and I do not recommend you do any of the things we did or that you necessarily follow any of the advice I give. I will give some advice, and I have some strong opinions, but I will tell you now that we did not follow our doctor's instructions 100%. We didn't feel it was necessary and felt like our doctor's orders were very overcautious. My father felt the same way about his surgery, and he didn't always follow all the rules either.

Please do not take our deviation from doctor's orders as permission for you to do the same. We took a risk in doing so. We are human, and humans cheat, lie, and do things they know aren't the best for them because we rationalize it will be ok. I took our health into our own hands by deviating, even slightly, from the doctor's recommendations. Should you feel compelled to do the same, even if you're compelled by something you read in this book, your health is your own responsibility.

Bariatric surgery is a big, scary animal. It's dangerous, even though it's routine. Don't be fooled by my writing style, which tends to be sarcastic and irreverent, especially in this case. Just because it worked for us doesn't mean it will work for anyone else.

Treat what follows as a fun story, journey, and anecdote... not as an example to follow. Your results may vary, some restrictions apply, only valid where not prohibited by law, past performance no guarantee of future results, provided 'as is' without any warranties expressed or implied, and, most importantly, read at your own risk.

Chapter 7

An Office Full of Taters

At first, we thought our nutritionist was a psychopath. Not literally, of course, but in that, "Hey, I'm totally crazy, and I live in a different world than the rest of humanity… so buckle up!" kind of way.

We decided to start seeing her because we knew from my father that seeing a nutritionist and being on a diet was a requirement for bariatric surgery. It was also a requirement for our insurance company to cover the procedure, so we figured we may as well start there. In the beginning, our only desire was to 'test the waters' and see how the diet thing would go. I was hoping we could lose the weight with diet alone. I mean, if we could avoid having surgery, then let's do that, and, if not, then we'd have the necessary nutritionist requirements checked off when it came time.

I wasn't looking forward to going. I had been to a nutritionist when I was in high school, and I thought I pretty much knew the routine. We'd go in, they'd tell us we're fat and that we need to stop eating so damn much of so damn many of the wrong things. We would sigh and agree. We would schedule another appointment, and 30 days later, would basically do the exact same thing all over again. I did not have much faith.

There was a small glimmer of hope, though. I thought, "Maybe they've discovered something great since the last time I went, or maybe we can just eat less of the stuff we like. I think I can live with only eating a small fry at McDonalds, instead of a large."

This, of course, was a stupid thing to think.

We made our appointment for the end of June 2016. As I said, we decided to go with the same bariatric and weight loss center that my father had used. Even though his experience was less than stellar, as far as the office was concerned, we really didn't go through the details with him and didn't know the specifics, only that the office was a pain in the ass. We rationalized a couple of things. First, the surgeon had changed in that office. We thought, "Well, if the surgeon is different, then the office probably runs differently, so we won't have the same experience Dad did." Second, we figured Dad's experience was probably an isolated event and had to do with Medicare or any of the other complications that Dad's specific situation had to offer, like changing insurance companies mid-stride or even his age.

As the appointment date grew nearer, we found ourselves going out to eat more. I've always been fond of going out to restaurants. I've always been fortunate enough to be able to afford it. There was a time when a co-worker and I would go out for lunch every day, and then I would also go out for dinner four or five times a week on my own. Once I was married, those things changed a little, mostly due to budget, but I still went out to lunch two to three times a week with my friend and out to dinner two or three times with my wife.

Our thought was that we've only got so long before the big bad nutritionist tells us we can't eat that good stuff anymore, and we better pack it in while we still have a chance. We went to all our favorite places in the weeks leading up to our first visit. As the time for our appointment grew nearer, my mood grew darker. Throughout the rest of the process, all the way up to the month before surgery, a nutritionist appointment would ruin my week because I would be dreading it. I hated answering for my 'food crimes.' That only changed late in the process, when I became absolutely forced to follow strictly the diet they had given me. I'll talk more about that later.

In the meantime, the date of our first appointment had finally arrived. Amanda and I went together. We figured we would go through the process together; that way, we could be on the same diet and support each other as we went through. Everyone thought it was a good idea, including the doctors and nurses, but that doesn't mean they made it easy. At first though, it kinda was. They let us schedule together and even go back to see the doctor together. We weighed in together and saw the nutritionist together.

The bariatric center is in a large building next to the main hospital. The medical plaza, as it's called, houses offices and clinics for many of the outpatient and diagnostic services the hospital provides. We would come to know this building very well in the year and a half that would follow.

We were both a bit nervous. Neither of us knew what to expect. We understood our eating habits would need to change after the visit, and that was about all we knew for sure. Secretly, I think, both of us hoped the visit would be basic and mostly tell us to stop eating restaurant food and watch our calories. Maybe add some exercise. We both felt like we could handle that. We had been psyching up for this for about a month and had gone through, what we thought, was every conceivable permutation of advice the nutritionist would give us. We felt as ready as we could be, given that we really had no idea what to expect. The nutritionist we were seeing was different than the one Dad had seen, and while Dad did meet our nutritionist once in a support meeting, the only thing he'd told us when we mentioned her was, "Yeah, I remember that lady." He may or may not have shuddered after he said that. Either I don't remember or have blocked it out.

We entered the office and signed in. It looked like every doctor's waiting room you've ever been in, except it had a glass cabinet with big bags of bariatric protein powder prominently displayed like trophies in a trophy case. There were strict signs about no cell phone use, which completely ignored by everyone, and the seats were ever so slightly, but not terribly, uncomfortable.

The receptionist called us up to the front window and did the sign in procedure. We had a stack of paperwork to fill out, and we each had our copay to take care of. So began the never-ending march of paperwork and bills. Had I known then what I know now, I may have had the check we wrote that day framed with a plaque that read, "The first $45 I ever gave to the bariatric center." It certainly would not be the last.

We both agreed later that the receptionist had the personality of a baked potato.

To be fair, the mood of the entire office for the first visit we had was just... terrible. Everyone seemed to be going through the motions. It was noticeable enough that my wife and I ended up making fun of the whole experience to all our friends. Sometimes, I think that was the best thing to come out of that entire visit. In any case, we certainly didn't expect that kind of a feeling from a visit to the nutritionist. I'm not sure what we expected, but we thought it would be more like, "Welcome to your new weight loss journey! We're glad you've finally decided to take control of your life and make the right decisions for your heath. Congratulations, let's get started!" And less like, "Yeah. You're fat. We can see that. Waddle your ass in here, so we can prove it and tell you what you can't eat anymore."

After waiting the requisite amount of time, which always seems to be much longer than you expect, our names were called. We waddled back into a small room, where a nurse told us to take off our shoes and socks for our weigh in. They had a fancy sort of scale that sends electricity through your feet and can tell how much bone mass, water, muscle mass, and fat you have, and probably could tell you my credit score.

The nurse was not cheery. She was not mean either; she was just... baked potato. I can't think of any other way to say it. When I took my socks off, though, she did blink to life for long enough to chastise me, "Ankles a little swollen today, are they?"

In my head, I raged, "Look lady, yeah, I'm a fatass, ok? I know I'm a fatass. That's why I'm here. Instead of mocking me and making me feel worse about myself, why don't you do your job and either shut the hell up or send me some encouragement?" Out loud, I said, "Oh... I hadn't noticed."

Once we were both weighed in and had all our vital signs checked, we were taken back to another waiting room. If you've ever been to the doctor, you know how this goes. You wait in the main waiting room until you're about ready to scream, then someone calls your name, and you can finally come back to get your vitals done. Then, once they've figured out how the blood pressure cuff works and get your life score sorted, they shuffle you off to yet another waiting room, where you wait for the actual doctor to get done playing chess with his old high school buddies or whatever the hell he's doing in there, so he can come knock on your door and smile like they haven't kept you waiting for an hour longer than you expected.

Eventually, the nutritionist came in to check us over. She listened to us breathe, checked our hearts, and rubbed our necks to check for swelling, I think. After that, she led us to her office. The first real sign of life we saw in the bariatric center that day, she was a nice, petite, and pretty lady in her 30's. She had a very nice smile and seemed like she was truly ready to help. Finally, I thought, a voice in the darkness. Someone I can trust. Someone I can relate to.

Whooo boy, was I wrong.

Chapter 8

The Caveman of Unsound Mind

The more the nutritionist talked, the more Amanda and I realized we were about to get into something completely unlike any diet we had ever heard of. Our conversation with the nutritionist started simply enough. She asked us what our eating habits were like, properly scolded us for eating poorly, told us our lives were going to need to change if we wanted to lose weight, all the stuff we expected.

When it came time to talk to her about what kinds of things we ate, we were honest. That may have been a mistake. As I said, the few weeks before our visit to the nutritionist, we acted like a couple of convicts enjoying our last meals. We knew our eating habits were bound to change, so we enjoyed all our favorites. Why not? Surely, the nutritionist would understand.

"You had what? Taco Bell? Oh Edwin, Taco Bell isn't even meat! McDonalds?! There isn't a single thing in that restaurant you should be eating. In fact, I don't think there is a single restaurant in this whole town that I would say is ok. They all cook their food in disgusting types of fat and most won't honor a request to cook food in 'good' fats. You need to be in charge of that by cooking at home."

She went on to tell us it was no wonder we were overweight, considering our diets, and even though there were some choices we were making that were ok, almost everything we were doing was wrong. The more we told her about what we ate, the more fault she found. The truly annoying part for me was that I knew what we were doing wasn't good for us; that's why we went to the damned nutritionist in the first place. The last thing I needed was to be chided over something I already knew I was doing wrong. At least, that's how I felt.

When I asked about having lunch at work with my co-workers and business meetings, I may as well have been talking to a brick wall. She told me I would just need to bring in my own food to the restaurant, and if they wouldn't allow that, well, I'd just have to stop going to lunch meetings. I told her that wasn't possible, and she told me I obviously didn't care enough about my health to make it possible. I was pretty well flabbergasted by that point, but I hadn't heard anything yet.

She asked us if we knew what a carbohydrate was. We said that we thought we did. She explained that carbs were found in breads, rice, potatoes, pasta, cereals, granola, and basically everything everywhere that isn't meat or fat. She then told us that we had to eliminate all the carbs from our diet. From this moment forward, we would no longer be allowed to eat any of those high carb foods, and what little carbs we could have every day had to come from vegetables. When I told her I didn't like vegetables, feeling for all the world like a man drowning in some kind of ocean of craziness, she told me I just wasn't preparing them correctly, and I needed to add more butter.

Somehow, butter was her answer for everything. If you don't like it, add butter! Not filling enough? Not enough butter! Or maybe heavy cream. Or bacon. Fat! Add fat! So much fat! Fat is good, fat is great, just keep adding fat. In fact, we want you to have more fat than protein. Fat should be the number one source of calories.

It turns out that my wife and I had stumbled into the paleo diet.

Our nutritionist explained it like this: See, tens of thousands of years ago, when mankind was still living in caves and choosing wives by bashing them over the head with a club, man didn't have the luxury of fresh baked muffins or glazed donuts. Man ate meat. Fatty meat, apparently. That's what our bodies are designed to handle, high amounts of protein and fat. Now that we all live in the lap of luxury and people want instant food gratification, all our food has become processed and loaded with carbs and sugar. Man was never meant to eat that much sugar so... diabetes and fatness everywhere. I'm pretty sure she looked at me when she said that.

In order to fix this epidemic of fatness, man needs to go back to the olden days, minus the hitting women over the head bit. My wife and I would need to cut carbs from our diet completely and focus on protein and, most of all, fat. Good fat, mind you. None of this yummy deep-fried vegetable oil stuff, but things like coconut oil, butter, and fatty meats. Bacon was our new best friend. Things that we had heard to stay away from our entire lives were suddenly a main focus of our diet.

In counterpoint, many of the things we had always heard to eat to stay healthy were now forbidden. Fruit, for one thing. We could no longer have fruit. In an effort to start eating healthier, I had recently begun having an apple as part of my lunch, rather than a bag of chips. I figured I would bring that up to the nutritionist when I got the chance... show that I was making an effort. No dice. As far as she was concerned, an apple was almost as bad as a bag of chips. Both were full of carbs. And carrots? I love carrots with ranch dipping sauce. Her view? The sauce is fine if it's high fat, but the carrots are terrible. Full of sugar. No more carrots.

Suddenly, my worst fears had come true. What I felt beforehand must be the worst-case scenario was actually happening. All the foods I really love, the ones I think about and fantasize about, and the ones I look forward to all day long were not simply reduced but completely eliminated. Before the nutritionist visit, I told myself I could handle reducing my portion sizes or cutting some fast food joints. I could start doing exercise or eating more vegetables, but to remove carbs entirely? To eat vegetables at every meal and make them my only source of carbohydrates? Then, to add insult to injury, the few vegetables I did like, such as corn or carrots, weren't allowed because they had too many carbs even for vegetables!

To say our heads were spinning a little bit is understating it. Part of me wanted to know if cavemen weren't allowed to eat fruit or carrots either, but I felt so knee deep in bizzaro world that I guess I forgot to ask. Amanda did ask about exercise though, and the answer didn't help our confusion. The answer was: don't.

What? Don't exercise? How much further down this rabbit hole can we go, doc? Next, you'll be telling us that up is down, left is right, and owning a leather jacket doesn't automatically make you cool. Her explanation for no exercise was that, apparently, studies show exercise doesn't help you lose weight. It helps you keep weight off that you have lost, but it doesn't help with weight loss. Besides, she wanted to make sure the diet was going to work for us, so she didn't want to add a variable like exercise. That those two things directly contradicted each other was not lost on me.

Next, we were given our marching orders. We were to download an app to our phones designed to keep track of our daily food intake and help us count our carbs, fats, protein, and calories. Not that the nutritionist cared about calories. In fact, she didn't care how many calories we ate in a day, so long as we stayed below 50 grams of carbs. That may not sound too hard, but that's three slices of bread, half a plate of pasta, or about a cup of rice. Keep in mind that almost everything has carbs in it, and if you buy anything pre-processed or, heaven forbid, from a fast food place, the carb count is going to be astronomical.

The nutritionist showed us how to use the app on her phone. It was all very easy and seemed simple enough. I, who had already done a tracking style diet in high school, wasn't impressed. Oh, it was nice that the phone did all the work, but suddenly, I was going to be accountable for all the things I ate, all the time. I hated it. I understood why it was important and still do, of course, but that doesn't change how I felt.

Once all of this was over and Amanda and I were properly shell-shocked, the nutritionist asked us if we thought we were going to be interested in getting bariatric surgery done, eventually. Looking back, it could almost be part of a scripted dance. Not that I think it was planned that way, but it was almost like, "Now that I've shocked you into submission and you're reeling with all this new information, it should be obvious to you that there's no way you'll succeed on this diet. Therefore, I'm obligated to suggest that you strongly consider bariatric surgery so that, when you fail, and you will, you still have an option to become the newer, healthier, you."

We told her it was an option, but we'd like to try the diet first. She agreed that was a good idea but suggested we each do a sleep study to determine if we have sleep apnea. Sleep studies were required by our insurance, as well as the bariatric office, before patients could undergo bariatric surgery, so she said it would probably be good to go ahead and get them done. They are a lengthy part of the process to have surgery and getting them out of the way would help if we decided to become surgical patients. As part of this, she asked each of us sleep related questions, such as, "Do you snore?" And, "Do you feel tired during the day?" My answers were pretty much yes, and "What? I'm sorry, I was dozing."

The nutritionist wasn't the first doctor of mine to suggest I should do a sleep study. Even my dentist had done so. Apparently, my gums looked like I was a mouth breather at night, so he asked if I snored. I told him that I did, according to my wife, and he said I should consider having a sleep study done. My family doctor had recommended it as well. I had always brushed it off as something old people do, and I certainly didn't want one of those stupid machines, so I never did one.

I guess now I would have to suck it up and get it done. Both of us would. I was not looking forward to it.

After she had written the orders for our sleep studies, she also gave us orders for blood work. The blood work would ensure we were getting the proper amount of vitamins and verify there wasn't anything else going on that would make this type of diet do more harm than good. I doubt cavemen had the luxury of lab tests, so I didn't expect there could be much that would show on blood work to prevent us from being on the diet.

At the end of the visit, we had all our orders, folders full of pamphlets and documents explaining how cavemen ate, and heads full of information we weren't sure we believed. We made our one-month follow-up appointment and left the medical plaza trying to rationalize what we'd just experienced. We told each other that we'd give it a try. Certainly, I admitted, it would be good for my diabetes. Plus, we thought, we both love bacon. Who doesn't? Bacon is awesome. Bacon, butter, cheese, fat, meat… yeah, we can do this. We had a lot to think about and a lot to plan.

We started coming up with meal ideas that didn't have any carbs. Things like meatloaf, hamburgers with no bun, pan fried chicken in coconut oil, and armadillo eggs would become staples. Armadillo eggs, if you didn't know, are jalapeños with the stem end cut off, de-seeded, stuffed with cheese and cream cheese, and then wrapped in bacon and grilled or baked. They're pretty amazing. We started talking about side-salads with the dressings we liked and what kind of vegetables I can tolerate.

For some reason, almost all the vegetables I like, I only like raw. I love raw broccoli dipped in ranch or raw celery topped with peanut butter. Luckily, both of these were on the new diet, so between them and side salads, which I like, I figured I'd be able to make it work. For my wife's part, she loves any kind of squash, green beans, asparagus, steamed broccoli, cabbage, or side salad, so the veggie part was going to be easier for her.

We talked about this on the way out of the building, and by the time we got to our vehicles in the parking lot, we were feeling a little better. We felt like we might be able to handle this thing. Each of us decided we'd get on Pinterest and start looking for good low carb recipes and see what we could find, but first, we had to get this tracking application the nutritionist had showed us.

We both downloaded the app then I went and had lunch at McDonalds.

Chapter 9

Cauliflower Dreams

For the next month or two, we gave it our version of the old college try. I talked to Dad about the diet, and he told me that, even though the surgeon and nutritionist were different, the office had basically put him on the same kind of diet as they did us. He agreed with us that 50 grams of carbs per day was a little on the restrictive side, so he just made sure he was less than 100 per day and called it good.

We took that piece of information and began to sculpt a new type of weekly menu for ourselves. I knew there was no way we were going to be 100% faithful to what the nutritionist had said; after all, we still thought she was crazy, but we got where we felt we were pretty close. We stopped going to restaurants during the week. When I went to lunch meetings with co-workers, I made sure to order things like hamburgers with no buns and a side salad instead of french fries. I found that having a taco salad without beans and tomato was fine, and as long as I didn't eat too much of the shell, I didn't feel guilty.

It wasn't what I would call amazing, but it was tolerable. After all, we did like a whole lot of the stuff on the diet. Steak was always a good choice, as was meatloaf, unbreaded fish, unbreaded chicken, pork ribs, brisket, pulled pork, and pretty much any kind of hamburger. Cheese was always a winner, and just about any kind of full fat sauce you could think of was perfectly ok. Cooking with lots of butter and fat was an adjustment, but we got used to it.

Sam's Club became a much more frequent stop for us. We would purchase huge blocks of butter and cream cheese, along with big bags of salad, stacks of hamburger patties, and bulk packages of bacon. We also stocked up on peanut butter, jerky, and pork rinds. Amanda doesn't like pork rinds, but I do. Or did, anyway, before the diet.

For the next few weeks, we were awash in a full fat meaty paradise. Not having potatoes or fruits didn't seem to matter that much when you can have the kind of meat and full fat stuff we were having. We felt mostly satisfied by every meal and were going through our bacon reserves quickly. Vegetables, it turns out, become much better when paired with bacon and fried in bacon grease.

It wasn't long, though, before there was trouble in caveman heaven. Foods that I loved, had loved my whole life, were now a very common part of my diet. They began to lose their luster. Pork rinds, once a treat, became an everyday sort of mundane replacement for chips. Celery and peanut butter, a fond friend of my childhood, began to feel like an unwelcome compromise for a snack cake. Bacon became the thing we added to everything to make it taste better, and even a food so beloved as the aforementioned armadillo eggs started to make our taste buds yawn, rather than cheer.

The upside to the diet was that weight loss did occur, for me anyway. Amanda never really saw any benefit, but my own weight dropped about ten pounds over the course of the first two months we were on the diet. I never knew why Amanda didn't lose the weight, other than the fact she's a woman and the cruel truth is that women have a harder time of it than men do. Even being seven years younger than me, it was still harder for her to lose weight.

My regular physician also had some good news for me during this period; my A1C had dropped. If I remember correctly, my A1C during that visit was 6.3. For a diabetic, 6.3 is very well-controlled, and my doctor even suggested I stop taking the sitagliptin since the diet was treating me so well. I readily agreed, considering sitagliptin was costing me over $100 a month. I felt good about myself, and even though the diet was starting to get old, I had a few good reasons to keep it up.

Even so, we yearned for the good old days of McDonald's hamburgers and Church's Chicken, as many of our favorite foods felt less and less appealing. We started saying things like, "Oh, what I wouldn't give for a piece of pizza." Or, "I'd love to just be able to go to Subway and have a foot long." We knew those things were forbidden, but in a strange way, that made them more appealing, not less. Soon after that, one of us floated the idea of a 'cheat day,' and it was instantly and unanimously decided that Saturday would be our new cheat day. On Saturday, we could have all the foods we normally couldn't. We rationalized that we would be good the rest of the week. After all, we deserved it for being so good! Hadn't I dropped my A1C level and lost weight? Sure, and since Amanda wasn't losing weight either way, what difference did it make for her?

Oh, how I looked forward to Saturdays during that time. We carefully chose what restaurants we would go to. If there were local places that we liked but didn't always have good stuff, like the local buffets, then we avoided them for fear that we would waste a meal on them. It was glorious. We truly appreciated the foods we ate that day in a way we never had before.

During the rest of the week, we brooded, waiting for Saturday. Getting desperate for a different kind of side dish, we remembered that our nutritionist had recommended mashed cauliflower as a substitute for mashed potatoes. Other places we read about it, and even some people we knew, confirmed it's actually very good. We decided to give it a try.

There are no words that I can write here that would express our disappointment with mashed cauliflower. It was awful. The taste, texture, and consistency were absolutely nothing like mashed potatoes, and trying to compare mashed cauliflower to mashed potatoes is the work of a demented soul, hell bent on salvaging something of the life they once knew.

We both hated it, Amanda more so even than I did, and that's saying something. We tried it twice; the second time we added enough butter to sponsor a college student in Wisconsin, and it still tasted terrible and felt like wet sand in our mouths. I actually found myself beginning to harbor animosity towards anyone with the audacity to say mashed cauliflower is 'just like' mashed potatoes… those people had fooled me into a false hope, and I could never forgive them.

Yet, we didn't learn. By the time we failed the second time on mashed cauliflower, our weekly regimen had become so stale that, food wise, Saturday was the only thing we had to look forward to. Sure, we still enjoyed some meals during the week. We didn't hate no-bun hamburgers or meatloaf yet, but they were dull. No excitement. For a couple of folks who spent their entire lives relishing their next meal and looking forward to what sort of food experiences may lie before them, having such a mundane and tired menu started wearing on us.

We started turning to places like Pinterest and Google, looking for ways to spice up our weekday menu. We found a plethora of low-carb breads, pizza crusts, and substitutes. Each one we found gave us hope that maybe, just maybe, we could find joy in the same kind of food we once ate by using its low or no carb counterpart.

We tried cauliflower and almond flour pizza crust. Crushing and crumbling the cauliflower into a thick paste and trying to wring every last bit of moisture out of it in a feeble attempt to make the final product even resemble something from a pizza place, or even a store bought frozen pizza, was a completely lost cause. No amount of wringing, drying, mixing, and baking could turn that cauliflower mush into something we didn't abhor putting in our mouths. Meals in which we tried to make it work turned into nothing but cheese and topping meals where the crust, if you can call it that, slid unceremoniously into the garbage, where it belonged.

When no amount of baking would suffice to get cauliflower into an edible form, we made what we considered our very last attempt at a cauliflower substitute for real food:

cauliflower grilled cheese. I reasoned with myself that, if you fry it in a skillet with some oil, anything will become crispy. My wife rationalized that adding enough cheese to anything will make it good enough to eat.

We were both wrong. Somehow cauliflower is cursed in our household. Everything we make with it turns to garbage, and, in all honesty, we can attribute more meals at Subway during our diet to failed cauliflower experiments than anything else.

The whole experience turned out to be extremely frustrating, and it began to sour us on the idea of substitution for foods we used to love. I started hating bloggers and recipe sites that proclaimed a certain type of carb-free bread or pizza crust was 'as good as the real thing,' or, heaven forbid, better. Amanda and I had many a night when we lamented to each other and griped heartily about people on the internet saying these substitutions are as good as the real thing.

"Are they stupid?" I would ask. "I mean, do they really believe that? How long has it been since this lady has had a real pizza?" It pissed me off, quite literally, that people would so casually spout such lies. It would be one thing if the recipe said, "Well, this isn't pizza crust, but it's the best you're going to get if you can't have carbs." No! They said things like, "Amazing cauliflower pizza crust! Better than the real thing! My family loves it, and yours will too!"

How dare they lure me in and give me such false hope that maybe, just maybe, they found the secret to making cauliflower taste like pizza dough, instead of the inside of an elephant's ass! I wasted my time on this recipe, bought the ingredients, spent hours cutting, mashing, drying, and baking the cauliflower only to throw away all that work in a disappointed haze.

And it wasn't just cauliflower. We found many, many recipes online that proclaimed to have the secret to making low-carb pizza crust, or bread, or biscuits, and every one of them was an exercise in disappointment. It wasn't long before we didn't trust any low-carb recipes we found on the internet. The more they shouted about how close to the real thing it was, the less we believed it.

The worst part of all of it, for me, was the buildup and disappointment. Every recipe said it was a replacement for something else. Everyone said it was 'just like' something else. Had the recipe been honest and said, "This is the no-carb version of a biscuit. It's not a real biscuit, but it's kind of the same." It wouldn't have been so bad. Every recipe we found ourselves comparing to the original food we tried to replace, and every one was sorely lacking.

It makes sense, now that I think back on it. If you really could make a far healthier version of pizza crust that tasted just like the real thing, pizza places would be offering cauliflower crust pizzas all over the place.

There's a reason they aren't.

The closest thing we found to actual pizza crust, and bread in general, was using almond flour and a huge amount of mozzarella cheese. Interestingly enough, if you mix almond flour with melted mozzarella, you can roll it into something not completely unlike pizza dough. You can then bake it and top it just like a real pizza.

It's not crisp, and it isn't doughy like pizza dough, but it's not bad for having zero carbs. It's very cheesy and a different kind of flavor, but as long as you don't try to pretend like it's pizza crust… it's pretty good.

We did find a few recipes that made us happy. We found that chicken in a batter made with coconut flour, fried in coconut oil, tasted quite good. As long as our carb limit was 50 grams a day, those didn't put us over budget. Wonton wrappers, also, didn't put us over budget if we baked some cream cheese and crab or jalapeno wontons. We started finding soups we enjoyed, especially a version of green chile chicken enchilada soup we found. It was a little bit of a cheat, since it contained beans, but the rest of the recipe contained no carbs whatsoever, so we let it slide. Again, under 50 grams a day.

We made a trip to Phoenix during this time and found a restaurant that sold low carb bread on one of our cheat days. The restaurant, Chompie's, is amazing, and their low carb bread is very good. It's not the same as real bread, but it's great for sandwiches. It's got a bit of a spongy texture, but the taste and usability for sandwiches more than makes up for it. If we could, we would get it all the time. Unfortunately, Chompie's is only in Phoenix. Having it shipped is far too costly, so we do without.

We didn't make one of our greatest discoveries until almost right before we had surgery. We found a low-carb quesadilla recipe online that called for something called 'Lavash Bread,' and we grabbed a package at the local Wal-Mart. Turns out, lavash bread is excellent, and a whole sheet of it is only 18 carbs. One sheet is easily enough to fold over and make an entire quesadilla, probably bigger than a standard sized tortilla. It comes out of the package soft, but crisps very easily and is tasty for being low carb. Amanda and I wish we would have found this much earlier in our diet.

Even with some success and a few good recipes to tide us over, though, we both knew the diet was going to fail eventually. We just couldn't sustain it. We found ourselves putting off our nutritionist visits and getting cranky with each other when one was coming up. We knew we'd get yelled at for our cheat day.

When we finally kept an appointment, our nutritionist did chastise us for having a cheat day. She told us the diet they put us on only works if we keep up with it, and cheating, even one day, somehow resets our body. If we cheat, we spend the next three days trying to get back into some kind of fat burning mode, and by cheating one day every week, we spent most of our time not burning fat.

I think each of us knew the diet was over at that point. We continued to try and continued to have cheat days. Instead of just Saturday, we did Saturday and Sunday. At different points throughout the next eight months, we would swing from trying hard to not trying at all. I will say we did adjust eating habits permanently as a result of our trial and error. All our meals were less carbs, and we stopped having bread with meals and having buns with burgers, brats, and hot dogs, but those were things we felt we could live with.

For my part, I was a bit angry. "If she thinks I'm never going to have french fries again, she's got another thing coming." I'd say, "I'd rather die early and enjoy my life than eat this crap and live an extra few years."

Privately, to ourselves, I think we both knew the ultimate outcome would be bariatric surgery. We needed time to prepare for that mentally, and it became just another reason to stray from the diet. After all, if I was going to spend the rest of my life eating like a bird, then I'd spend my last full-stomached summer enjoying myself, dammit.

Chapter 10

Sleepin' Ain't Easy

My sleep study happened first, and then, about a week later, Amanda had hers done. Before we could lay down and sleep for an audience, though, we had to go see a sleep doctor that could confirm we were, in fact, fat and needed to do a sleep study. We made our appointments and paid our co-pays for the privilege, which seems to be customary for anything health related. The sleep doctor was nice, but, like many of the doctors we would see in the coming months, very brief.

I've never understood how a doctor can charge you somewhere between $20 and $60, depending on your insurance, and spend an incredible two or three minutes with you to tell you something you already know. This is, of course, after they've had you poked and prodded by their underlings and after they've made you wait long enough to watch an episode of Cheers. Once they do show up, they give you just a few minutes before they vanish like a sock in a clothes dryer. You're then left with their underlings again to make a follow-up appointment. That appointment will also cost you the co-pay of $20-$60. In the meantime, they've billed your insurance something like $200 to $600 just so they could talk to you for less time than a beer commercial during the Super Bowl.

It's times like those when I feel as though maybe I'm in the wrong business.

As I said, the sleep doctor was nice but brief. I can pretty much sum up what she said like this, "Ok Mr. Edwin, because of your weight, it's very likely you have sleep apnea. We're going to schedule a sleep study to determine this. Please make an appointment with the front desk for next week. Have a nice day." The only other thing I remember was how she felt sure I was a surgical patient. At that time, Amanda and I were simply trying to use the diet for weight loss and hadn't decided on the surgery. When I told the doctor this, she seemed disappointed, "Well, when you eventually do have the surgery (because you're a fat ass who can't stick to a diet... I've seen this before), it's likely any sleep apnea you have will resolve on its own after you've lost weight, so that's good news."

I just so happened to be the last sleep study patient fortuitous enough to spend the night in an actual hospital room. After me, all sleep study patients would be placed in a new out-patient facility built next to the hospital. They were even in the process of moving things out while I moved in for the night. Not that it mattered. It turns out that trying to sleep during a sleep study is equally stupid and aggravating, no matter where you sleep, unless it's at home.

I arrived at the hospital at my designated time and went up to where my room for the night was supposed to be. Essentially, it looked like any other corridor in a hospital, dreary and sterile. The room was a disguised patient room. The bed wasn't a hospital bed, but everything else about the room was hospital standard, right down to the itty-bitty television with the weird combination nurse call / bed control / TV remote. On my way in, I talked to the 'sleep technician' in charge of the sleep study corridor. He told me to go ahead and settle into the room. Apparently, he had other folks to turn into human computer consoles before he got to me.

If you've never done a sleep study, you may not understand what I mean when I talk about turning folks into computer consoles. The number of wires hooked up to a person during the study is staggering. I felt like I was in a cheesy low-budget version of *The Matrix*. Once my time came, the technician asked me to change into my sleeping clothes. Fortunately for us both, I read the documentation for the study that pleasantly, but firmly, requested that I not plan on sleeping in the nude. I donned my sleeping attire, a simple t-shirt and workout shorts, and waited for the technician to return. Being a web developer who writes computer code for a living, the idea of being wired up to a machine was pretty fascinating to me, so I was actually looking forward to seeing how this would play out.

When he finally returned, he had a wiring harness unlike anything I had seen in my life. He moved a chair to the center of the room and asked me to take a seat. Fascinated, I sat. He asked me to hold this strange looking box for him while he set about wiring me up. One by one, he plugged in the little wires to the box, and one by one they found themselves somewhere on my body. Over the next ten minutes, we carried out this intricate little dance where I would stand, sit, stand, fish wires, and, all the while, hold on to the little box. I had to run wires down through my shorts, up into my shirt, and all over my head. I think the worst part was the hair goo.

Oh, the hair goo. It deserves its own paragraph. Because they're measuring some super magical kind of brain stuff (I'm not a doctor), they have to hook these sensors up to your head as close to your brain as they can get. For someone who, luckily for me, still has a mostly full head of hair, that means they need some way of attaching said sensors to your scalp without shaving your head. They accomplish this with some kind of otherworldly goop that seems to be a liquid and a solid at the same time. The technician took two or three globs of the stuff, stuck them in my hair, and then subsequently stuck a wire to them. It's impossible to describe the consistency of this stuff with any accuracy. When I put my hand up there later to verify it wasn't chewing gum, the texture was like hair gel with the viscosity of Jif Peanut Butter. It didn't 'squish' like peanut butter though, and it didn't really stick to my hand. It felt like I could mold it, but only if I were determined to do so. All I know for sure is that I was relieved to be rid of it the next morning when I could finally take a shower. It took a bit, but hot water and shampoo, along with a vigorous scrubbing, made the goo finally relent and dissolve. I'm assuming it's now in my septic tank somewhere, plotting to overthrow the government.

At the beginning of the study, they asked me what my normal bed time was. Like a dumbass, I told the truth, 11 pm or thereabouts. Once I was all hooked up and ready to go, the technician told me I could watch television until my bed time. They didn't want to disrupt my normal routine, you know, besides the hospital room, hair goo, and dozens of wires. Once I was hooked up, I looked at the clock, which told me 9pm. Damn, now I had to sit and watch crappy hospital cable for two hours while the goo got used to living in my scalp and all those wires were hanging off my face. Perfect. To pass the time, I took a picture of myself and sent it to my wife, so she could see what she would be up against during her study.

Once my bedtime finally arrived, I was more than ready to get some sleep. The technician had one final procedure to put me through though, and that was a test of his equipment. He asked me to lie down on the bed, which was no small task with all the wires attached to the little box I was still holding, and then he took the box and hooked it up to a wire coming from the wall. I assumed this was a communication wire that led back to a console somewhere, and I was right. He left the room and went to his console. What it looked like I have no idea, but I like to imagine it looked like an evil lair with monitors all around and a cat gently purring away in the technician's lap.

He asked me to perform several tasks, such as breathing in and out, looking up, down, and side to side, moving my legs, and blinking my eyes. After each task, he would either tell me I did well or that I needed to do it again. He came back into the room and added a set of nasal cannulas to my ensemble, presumably in case I decided to stop breathing sometime during the night, and told me I was good to go. He finished by explaining it was common for folks to be given a CPAP machine in the middle of the night. This was so they could do what's called a 'split study,' meaning I would go one half without and the other half with a machine to gauge how well I did both ways. I remembered my father telling me about a split study too, since that's what happened to him. I asked the technician how they determine if that happens and he simply shrugged and said, "It depends."

Completely unsatisfied with that answer, I decided to let it go and get some sleep. Once the technician left the room, it was time for some shut eye. I felt confident it wouldn't take me long. At home, I usually fall asleep within ten to fifteen minutes, and while it takes me longer in a strange place, I rarely have difficulty falling asleep. The wires made it harder, but before I was put to bed, the technician had bundled them up like a techno pony tail flowing out from my head. In this way, the whole bundle could be manipulated and easily moved should I find the desire to toss and turn. I found out quickly the bed was uncomfortable, and, despite what you may think, a hospital is not a great place to find sleep.

Unfortunately, that was a very long night. I couldn't sleep, no matter how hard I tried. As the minutes bled into hours, I began to wonder if I would ever nod off. The longer the night got, the more I felt like a failure. I started questioning everything. I have sensors on my legs, so don't move them! They'll think you have restless leg syndrome and give you more forever medication. I wanted to know what time it was but looking at my phone seemed like a bad idea. Knowing the time felt like an admission of defeat, and we've all had that long night where, the later it gets, the harder it gets to go to sleep. I was afraid I'd start saying things to myself like, "It's only 1am. If you sleep now, you'll get six good hours." Then, "It's only 2. You can still get five hours." As it got later and later in the morning, I turned more and more desperate to get some shut eye.

I began to wonder what would happen if I didn't sleep. Would that invalidate the study? Would I need another one? Does that mean I'd get charged twice? How much is this costing me? Shouldn't he be in here with a CPAP machine by now? What time is it, anyway? What if I got up to look out the window? Would that show up on his console?

By sometime toward the end of the study, I think I managed a little sleep. It's hard to know, though. If I did, it's the kind of sleep where you're not sure if you're awake or sleeping. When the technician finally came in and turned on the light around 6am, I thought for sure it was about 3am and he was going to give me a machine. When he started unplugging things and made it clear my study was over, I finally looked at my phone to see the time. I asked him if I'd slept at all and he said, "Not much." I asked about the split study, and he said there wasn't enough data to do a split study, and the doctor would need to see the data and determine the next course of action.

I went home that morning tired, disappointed, and ready for a hot shower. I stopped at a fast food place on the way because I was hungry and felt like I deserved a cheat after the night I'd had. Thankfully, I took the day after my sleep study off work, so I had some free time. I met my wife on her way out the door and told her the bad news. She consoled me a bit, and I went off to shower and get cleaned up. Then I went to bed. I slept like the dead.

Chapter 11

Sleepin Still Ain't Easy

Amanda's results during her sleep study were far better than mine. She actually managed a few hours of shut-eye during her study. Luckily for her, that meant she could be diagnosed without a follow-up study. Unfortunately for me, I failed my die roll and had to do the whole thing again. My second study would be done in the new facility, just as Amanda's was, and I remained hopeful that I would fare better my second time.

The new facility looked nicer and felt more like a hotel room than a hospital, but it still somehow managed to have that clinical charm we all know and love from the medical community. It was in an outpatient building designed for things like sleep studies, blood draws, and other things that the hospital was tired of overseeing. The same sleep technician greeted me for my second outing, and the procedure was almost identical.

The technician informed me that the doctor, somehow, mulled out enough data from my first study to determine that I did, indeed, have sleep apnea. This meant I would be given a CPAP machine to sleep with. I was a little excited to try something new, but mostly worried that I would have even more problems falling asleep than last time because I now had a humongous mask-thing on my face blowing hurricane force winds down my throat.

Before I could do much more than settle in, the tech let me know the television hadn't been hooked up yet. He was sorry, but there wasn't anything he could do. I was sorry too. Crappy hospital cable is better than no cable at all and sitting there with my thumb up my butt for two hours would be more than a little annoying. Fortunately for me, I had the best in new-age entertainment right in my pocket, my cell phone. He also neglected to tell me that I could adjust the firmness of the air-bed in the room, or that I could modify the temperature by adjusting the thermostat. He didn't tell me the former because he forgot to. He didn't tell me the latter because it was impossible. Amanda discovered halfway through her night that she could adjust the firmness of the bed. I was glad to have the information beforehand and a bit perturbed the technician hadn't told either of us.

I settled in, got my night clothes on, got all hooked up to the Matrix, and set about entertaining myself. You would think playing solitaire on such a small screen for two hours would tucker me right out. By the time the lights went out and I did all the sanity checks for the technician in his little control room the second time, I should've been ready to travel blissfully to the land of nod, breathing like some kind of discount Darth Vader and generating gobs and gobs of beautiful sleep data. It didn't happen that way.

I'd tried my father's CPAP mask just for fun when he received his. I remember wondering how anybody could sleep with that thing blowing so much wind in your face. It was crazy. Taking the mask off caused an incredible whooshing and gushing sound and sealing it to my face made me feel like my lungs were going to explode and my eyes pop right out of my head. He told me he could no longer sleep without it, and it was something people got used to.

The mask I used during the study was nowhere near as powerful as my father's, but that didn't stop it from feeling like I was wresting the air flow all night. Breathing in wasn't bad. In fact, it was pleasant, minus the stupid mask on my face and the ridiculous hose wrapping itself around everything. Breathing out was another story. I felt like I had to muscle the air out of my lungs. Each breath out was a concerted effort in expelling the air I had so I could get more. Each breath in was a sweet relief from the exertion of fighting against the pressure until the air had to be breathed out, and then the fight was on again to get that old air the hell out of my body.

I fought all night to get into a rhythm where I could breathe without thinking. The harder I tried, the harder it was. Once you think about breathing, of course, you can't breathe unless you concentrate on it manually, and forcing each breath made me think about it constantly. Thinking about it constantly made me desperately want to stop thinking about it, which made me think about it more. Tossing and turning, wires sticking out of goo in my scalp, a techno pony-tail, a flight-suit mask, and a ridiculous air hose flopping around throughout it all became my stuff of nightmares.

I did not sleep. Again, I did not look at my phone, diligently refusing to give in to my desire to know the time. This time, when the technician arrived in the morning and turned the light on, I had an overwhelming sense of defeat and relief. I didn't bother to ask him if I slept. I knew the answer. I disconnected myself from the wiring harness, packed up my things, and walked silently out into the cool morning air. Again, I had a fast food breakfast because I deserved it.

The result of both of our tests came back that we both had sleep apnea. The sleep doctor tuned our machines to the data she had, which was a fair bit for Amanda and next to none for me. We each took our turn visiting a local medical equipment place that oversaw distributing the machines. We each received our machine and a mask, for which we were not offered a choice. Amanda's machine was set to a nice gentle breeze, barely perceptible when wearing the equipment. Mine was set to F3 tornado. My settings did have one redeeming quality, however. The machine automatically understood when I was breathing in vs when I was breathing out and adjusted itself to reduce the air flow when I wanted to exhale. This one simple feature made a world of difference.

It didn't take long for Amanda and me to get used to the machines. We were informed that failure to use the machines, which have a cell phone chip in them that phones home to tell on us if we're bad, would result in the insurance company not paying for them. That was enough to keep both of us honest and using the machines every night. It turns out that I felt better using the machine. I was less sleepy during the day, and I felt like I was less cranky. Amanda has told me she doesn't feel any different after using her machine, but her settings are so low that we suspect the sleep doctor of diagnosing her with sleep apnea, just so the hospital could make another buck. It's also one of the qualifying required medical conditions for bariatric surgery, so we thought that might have something to do with the diagnosis as well.

The bill for the CPAP machines wasn't too bad, considering what they do. Each of us had a bill of around $30 a month. Not that I enjoyed paying for something I had to wrestle with every night to go to sleep, but at least it wasn't bank breaking for us. The bill for the actual sleep studies was another story. Amanda was charged over $300, after insurance, by the hospital for her one night. I was charged almost $700 for my two nights. This is a charge from the hospital, not the sleep doctor that did the study. Her charges were around $100 and $200 for Amanda and me, respectively.

I was outraged when we received the bills. Outraged and confused. To be honest, I think the sleep study was the first time either of us had a procedure that carried a separate bill from both the doctor and the hospital. I now know this is typical, but at the time, I had no idea. Up to that point in my life, I'd never had to stay in a hospital or receive any treatment from different sources that billed separately, and I didn't know who to pay. I honestly thought we could ignore the hospital bills because the doctor bill should take care of it. When I called the doctor's office and asked, they confirmed the doctor's bill was the only bill I had to pay. Later, I realized that, as far as the doctor's office was concerned, their bill **was** the only bill I had to pay. They didn't care about the hospital's bill. The hospital, however, did care.

Calling the hospital confirmed I had to pay the doctor and the hospital separately. I was flabbergasted and a little distraught. Where was I going to come up with over a thousand dollars to pay these bills I didn't even plan for? Why the hell didn't the doctor tell me it was going to cost this much? How can they just expect us to pay this? How can they get away with not even telling us how much it's going to cost beforehand?

My wife and I firmly believe there is some sort of crazy epidemic in health care in this country that's almost entirely ignored by everyone. I'm not talking about Obamacare or any kind of healthcare reform. I'm not going to open that can of worms. No, what I'm talking about is the attitude that, "Your health is the most important thing, and cost is not a factor." The hell it isn't. Cost is a factor for everything for every person I've ever known in my life. I don't know anyone for whom cost is not a factor. Cost is not only a factor, it's the single greatest factor for a huge amount of the decisions we all make in everyday life. Should I get a steak or a hamburger? Cost is a factor. Should I buy a 4k TV or settle for 1080p? Cost is a factor. Should I buy a car or take the bus and pretend the smell isn't so bad? Cost is a factor.

Why is it that, when it comes to our health, cost is not a factor? In every interaction we had with a doctor, nurse, or other healthcare practitioner throughout this entire process, at no time did cost ever factor into any part of the decision making. They all just assumed, somehow, we could pay for everything, no matter the cost. In fact, they never even mentioned cost. It seems almost like a taboo subject in the doctor's office. If you ask about how much something costs, they blather on about how precious your health is and ask if you really want to attach a number to your health. This was never more apparent to us than during the sleep study. My father couldn't warn us either because he has Medicare, and it pretty much took care of it. He was as shocked at the cost as we were.

The sleep study was not the only time, early on, that the cost of something shocked us. One of the first trials we had to endure during our seemingly never-ending gauntlet of medical tests was blood work. The nutritionist ordered each of us to have blood work done so she could verify our health and look for any potential issues. No problem, I thought. I've had blood work done before. I'll just go in, they'll stick me, and it'll cost around $70-$80, maybe as high as $120, but blood work isn't that big a deal. I figured, between the two of us, we should get in for under $200. That's a bunch, but not enough to make a huge dent in our monthly cash flow, so we could absorb it.

I wasn't counting on the test for Vitamin D. I don't know the specifics, but apparently testing for Vitamin D requires either gold plated lab equipment or a trained monkey fueled by caviar and unicorn tears. When the blood tests were all said and done, Amanda was charged almost $300, and I was charged almost $400. As a side note, each of us were charged different amounts for almost everything throughout the process, which, to be honest, I still can't understand and don't care to investigate.

Just like the sleep study, which, at the time of the blood tests we hadn't even done yet, I was livid when we got the bills from the hospital. Why the hell didn't the nutritionist tell us how expensive it was going to be? We've done blood tests before, and they were nowhere near this expensive. During our next nutritionist appointment, we decided to ask her about it.

The response from the nutritionist was surprising. She was frustrated. "They told me they weren't going to charge our patients that much anymore! This isn't the first time this has happened; they shouldn't be that expensive. We negotiated with them to lower their prices for our patients." She told me to talk to the office manager, and they would get this all figured out for us.

Thus began a long and arduous process of trying to get ahold of the bariatric center office manager and, at the same time, fending off the bill collectors for the hospital. Several phone calls and months later, there was still no resolution, even though the office manager was adamant that she would take care of it for us.

In the middle of dealing with the blood work issue, the bills for the sleep study came in, and that only added fuel to my fire when it came to dealing with the hospital and money. By this time, we owed the hospital almost $2000 by their books, and I was desperate to find a way to deal with that incredible number. I began calling the hospital billing center in Tucson, a company farmed out by the hospital to deal with people like me. I was always nice to them on the phone, but I was also very firm and obviously angry.

They told me the best they could do was take 35% off my bills if I paid them all at once. That was better than nothing, and even though it didn't make me happy, I eventually agreed to those terms because Amanda and I were in the process of buying a new home, and I didn't want any kind of unpaid bill to ding our credit if it went into collections. Even though I paid the bills, I wrote a very long and detailed letter to the hospital regarding the conditions of the sleep study rooms and how I felt it was wrong to be billed so much for the terrible sleeping conditions. I noted the uncomfortable beds, lack of TV in the new facility, and the lack of information about basic comfort items in the room, such as the thermostat and bed firmness settings. I even claimed I felt the poor conditions of the first room in the hospital prevented me from getting any sleep, necessitating my second night. I argued I shouldn't even be billed for the second night because the only reason I needed it was because their hospital room sucked so bad.

I also mentioned, almost in passing, that we were also in negotiations about being overcharged for bloodwork. All in all, I argued, the whole situation pretty much made Amanda and me feel like we were being bent over the table and manhandled by a caviar addicted monkey. I sent the letter and called the billing office in Tucson. They told me they received it and would forward it to management. I never heard from the billing office again.

I did hear from the office manager for the bariatric center, who asked me if I'd ever made any progress with the bloodwork billing. When I told her no, she sighed heavily and told me she had talked to the actual hospital billing manager, not the Tucson call center but the actual person in town in charge of billing, and that person told her it would be taken care of. I asked for the hospital billing manager's number and got it. I now had in my possession the number of a real person in the town I lived in that had an actual office in the hospital, and I hoped that person could help me.

When I called and finally got ahold of her, she didn't have much time for me. She let me know she had heard some of the details but not all of them. She asked me to email her the specifics and gave me her email address. Solid gold, as far as I was concerned. I finally had a place at the hospital I could send correspondence and, hopefully, it wouldn't get lost in some endless billing bureaucracy. I re-drafted the letter I originally sent to Tucson billing and sent it to the hospital billing manager.

Probably a month or so later, after not hearing anything, she must've been going through her backlogged tasks and noticed she had one with my name on it. She sent me an email and asked what my story was and if I had any more details for her. I sighed and began re-drafting my letter again, hoping against hope that something would come out of it. As I was writing, another email came into my inbox. That email explained how she had found the email I sent months earlier and decided to refund our money for all three sleep studies, as well as both our bills for the bloodwork. She stated, "I didn't realize that you were so unhappy with our services and feel terrible that I missed that original email sent to Tucson with the aggravating details."

Again, I was flabbergasted, but this time, it was the happy version. Somehow through perseverance, firm anger, and a bit of hospital disregard, we had our money back. It took almost six months and an endless number of letters, emails, and phone calls, but we finally got back what we deserved and more. I'm glad we did, because eventually we would need it... to pay the hospital.

Chapter 12

Decisions, Decisions

On August 21ˢᵗ of 2017, the United States played host to its first total solar eclipse in almost 100 years. Certainly, it was the first total solar eclipse I had the means and the time to attend. A total solar eclipse is one of those things that, even though they aren't incredibly rare, most folks don't ever get to see, simply because they don't happen conveniently. Usually, a total eclipse happens somewhere over an ocean, or in some far-off country that is far too expensive, or dangerous, for an everyday joe like me to reach.

I made up my mind years beforehand that I wasn't going to miss the 2017 eclipse for any reason, no matter what. Since I'm married, that meant I also had to figure out how to convince my wife to tag along. Luckily for me, it wasn't too hard. She's nowhere near the astronomy buff that I am, but she knew it was important to me, and she knew, from my incessant prattling on about it, it was going to be one hell of a show.

We decided to spend the day of the eclipse in Casper, Wyoming. From my research, it seemed like the place to be… wide open spaces, great chance of clear skies, and not terribly far from home base in Las Cruces, New Mexico. We made a vacation out of it, and we felt incredibly blessed when the skies, and the wonderful folks in Casper, cooperated with our plans and presented us with one of the most spectacular sights I've ever seen in my life. I could write a whole other book about that experience. Who knows, I might.

We decided before we left that we would take the diet our nutritionist put us on and throw it right out the window. By the time of our eclipse trip, both of us knew deep down that surgery was going to be right around the corner. Up to that point, we hadn't formally discussed it, but the idea came up in random conversations from time to time, so it was no stranger.

Vacations are hard on diets. Going to a place with new food, in many cases amazing new food, puts a strain on even the most devout dieter. We were not that devout and knew we couldn't hold up against the caliber of fine dining options we would have throughout our trip. Instead, we rationalized that vacation would be our last hurrah before seriously talking about the surgery.

The food on our vacation was glorious. We went to a place in Jackson Hole that served a single plate with buffalo prime rib, elk steak, and venison sausage all in one go. I had that, while my wife had a buffalo spare rib plate. Other times, we visited fast food joints that didn't exist in New Mexico or partook in some local cuisine. We even ate some street food in Casper, while attending the festival. I had a non-diet huckleberry lemonade. I do not feel guilty.

Once we returned from our trip, we tried to get back on the diet horse, but our hearts weren't in it. Food, essentially, beat us. Powerless against it, we had our first serious talk about having bariatric surgery and decided it was time. If either of us were ever going to lose the weight, and if my wife was going to have a chance at pregnancy, we felt like we didn't have a choice. Knowing my father made the decision much easier because we could use his success as proof that it works.

We called the bariatric center and let them know. They set up another in a series of appointments with our nutritionist, this time to focus on the surgery. They didn't seem surprised. It seems diet alone is a long shot, and almost everyone who goes through their office opts for the surgery, eventually, if not right off the bat. In fact, as we would find out later, almost all the patients at the bariatric center start out looking for bariatric surgery, instead of even trying the diet first.

Months earlier, the bariatric center informed Amanda and me that we could no longer schedule our appointments together. They gave us some kind of jive about how scheduling two people together used up two appointment slots. They explained that, when folks going together canceled, they usually cancelled both slots. Two time slots being cancelled at the same time made for big problems or some such thing. Their new policy, then, was to allow two folks to schedule next to each other, but they had to see the doctor separately. I did not fight them or tell them how stupid that was. Two people scheduled back to back cancelling together would be worse than two people scheduled at the same time cancelling together, but I had my suspicions there was an ulterior motive. I had no idea what it would be and didn't really care.

It did make visiting the nutritionist a lot more awkward for us, though. We were trying to go through the process together, so we could support each other. If we could be in the same office, we could ask questions that both would gain the benefit from. Separating us made it so that we each had knowledge gaps. That wasn't really a big deal, but it also meant that, many times, we each saw a different nutritionist.

There were two nutritionists in the office, the head nutritionist doctor and her assistant. The assistant tended to be a bit less crazy and a bit less strict. Every time we went, we hoped we'd get the assistant, but the time we went to talk about the surgery, they split us up and put each of us with a different nutritionist. I got the assistant and Amanda got the doctor. Neither of them talked much about the surgery. Instead, they both admonished us on our food tracking and how we hadn't lost any weight. The assistant suggested I try fasting.

At the end, both of us, independently, asked about surgery requirements and changes to our diet. Both nutritionists told us there would be no changes to the diet, and they had 'navigators' to move us through the surgery procedures, so we wouldn't miss anything. We both, independently, wondered what the hell we needed to visit the nutritionist for anyway.

I made it to the navigator first. She sat in her own office, which had examples of protein power, protein drinks, and protein soups on a shelf. When I sat down, she didn't begin at the beginning, like I expected. Instead, she began somewhere in the middle by giving me a stack of paper work and asking if I'd been seeing the nutritionist for long.

I told her about a year. She said, "Oh, well then, you've met that requirement. You'll also need a sleep study, a psychological examination, an EKG, an EGD, and blood work." I told her I already had my sleep study done, and I already had blood work done too. "Good!" She said, "The sleep study takes the longest, so it's good that you've got that done."

My next question, in my mind, was the most important. I asked, "What are the chances of getting this done this year?"

She said, "Well, with your sleep study done, I would say… good."

"Good?" I asked. "Ok, because I want to make sure we do everything the same year. If there's a chance my wife and I can't get it done this year, we need to postpone it to next year. See, my insurance…"

"Oh, has she had her sleep study done?"

"Well, yes," I replied.

"Good. That's the longest part. If you've both had it done already, and you've both been seeing the nutritionist for over three months… has she?"

"Yes." I sighed.

"Good. Well then, you've both got most of the hard stuff out of the way. You should be able to get it done this year."

"Ok," I said, pressing this time. "Because if we get everything done this year, we'll both hit our max out of pocket and insurance can take care of the bulk of the bill, but if we do most of the testing this year and then have the actual surgery next year… our cost will double."

"Oh yes, I completely understand," she replied, dismissively. "All you have left…"

It was about that time my wife walked in the room. She finished her appointment with the doctor, and they decided to have us both see the same navigator. I was glad about that, but it meant the navigator had to go back through and re-explain everything Amanda had missed.

But she didn't. She just kept right on going.

"All you both have left is the psych exam, EKG (electrocardiography), blood work and the EGD (esophagogastroduodenoscopy). Then you should be all set," she said.

We told her, again, that we already had blood work done, and she seemed pleased with that. Before we left, she gave us a very quick overview of what we would need to do and how we would need to eat leading up to and following the surgery. We left her office with a few doctor's orders and a feeling of being run though the whole thing much too quickly. It was almost... anticlimactic. On our way out, we made an appointment with the actual surgeon to talk about options. Thus started our countdown to the end of the year and my new full-time job: worrying about how we were going to pay for it all.

Our surgeon's appointment was almost a month away, so we spent the next few weeks scheduling our other appointments. Each one went out further than the last. I began to worry about getting it all done before the end of the year.

When we went for our appointment with the surgeon, they decided to let us both see her at the same time for some reason. Maybe cancelling on a surgeon isn't as big a deal as cancelling on a nutritionist. In any case, I was glad. It meant both of us could ask questions and both of us would hear the answers.

Our visit with the surgeon was surprisingly short. She asked many of the same questions that every person in the office had asked up to that point and verified we were still alive (heartbeat, breathe in and out etc.). She went over the different surgery options and asked us which one we thought we wanted. We both told her we wanted gastric sleeve. She asked if we were sure. We were.

There are basically three types of bariatric surgery procedures we had access to: gastric sleeve, gastric bypass, and the lap-band. There are more options than this, but those three are what our surgeon would do, and from my own research, they are, by far, the three most popular weight loss procedures. What follows is my understanding of these three procedures, and that's probably not saying much.

The lap-band is a device the surgeon implants on the upper part of the stomach, just below where the esophagus and the stomach meet. It's literally a band that goes around the upper part of the stomach and creates what the surgeon called a stoma, which is just a way of saying opening. Basically, this creates a very small upper stomach pouch that restricts the amount of food that can be ingested at one time. The size of the stoma, and correspondingly the amount of food that passes through it, can be adjusted by inflating or deflating the band with a saline solution.

Of the three choices, the lap-band is the only one that is fully reversible. If a patient decides they don't like it, it can be taken out, and they'll pretty much go back to being the same as they were prior to the band's implementation. This is a benefit to some folks for whom the idea of permanent surgery is distasteful.

Far more distasteful to me, however, is that the lap-band requires the installation of a port in your abdomen for inflating and deflating the band if you need adjustment. The surgeon said the port would be under the skin, meaning that inflating and deflating the band would be done with a needle, but I still had no desire to have a port installed in my body. I've seen The Matrix and, thanks to the sleep study, already knew what that felt like.

I've also read that adjustments to the band put patients back at square one as far as liquid diets and growing accustomed to your new stoma size again, so that seemed like a pain in the ass I didn't want to deal with. Lap-band patients need constant maintenance, as well. Going to the doctor for an oil change every three thousand miles didn't seem like fun to me. Pass.

The second procedure, and the one my aunt had done in 1989, is the gastric bypass. Some people also call this the Y. During gastric bypass, the surgeon sort of disconnects a small thumb-sized portion at the top of the stomach from the rest of the stomach. This small portion is then sewn up to form a pouch, while the rest of the stomach is also sewn up to heal and continue creating gastric juice or whatever it does.

Once the new small pouch is created, the small intestine is cut just below where it attaches to the old stomach, and the lower portion of the now cut intestine is brought up and connected to the pouch. This is your new tiny stomach. The cut part of the intestine, below the old stomach, is connected to the moved portion of the intestine lower down. This is where the Y comes in because the small intestine now makes a Y with the new stomach pouch on the right side of the Y, and the old stomach on the left side, both connected to the small intestine.

This is called bypass because food essentially bypasses the bigger portion of the stomach and the first little bit of the small intestine. This has two benefits. First, the small stomach means you can't eat as much. Second, bypassing part of the small intestine means the food you eat doesn't get absorbed as much.

Because it restricts the amount you eat and reduces the amount of absorption, gastric bypass tends to have the highest success rate. With a stomach the size of a thumb, you have no choice but to eat very tiny amounts. If the goal is to lose weight, get rid of diabetes, and drastically change your life... the bypass is probably the right choice.

Unfortunately, the bypass does have some serious drawbacks, especially for me. One of the worst is called 'dumping syndrome.' Dumping syndrome is nasty. It's typically caused by eating too much sugar or carbs, and it happens because the pouch is so small and so close to the new small intestine connection that sugary food moves into the small intestine too quickly. When that happens, the body freaks out and tries to dilute the sugar with gastric content, dumping it into the intestines. What happens next sounds like the list of side effects on a bad medication commercial.

Bloating, diarrhea, dizziness, heart palpitations, nausea, vomiting, sweating, risk of farting in front of relatives, the list goes on and on. I'm sure I don't have to tell you, but vomiting is probably the scariest thing on that list, depending on your relatives. Vomiting after bariatric surgery is a special kind of hell. Like a sneeze, a chunder stresses your internal organs to the max. Unlike a sneeze, the maximum pressure while blowing chunks is focused on your stomach. You know, that thing you just had major surgery on... the one that's not healed yet and still has staples and stiches in it. That thing.

No thanks. I don't know about anyone else, but this guy still likes the occasional Twinkie and doughnut. Even after surgery, I planned to have half a Twinkie or quarter-doughnut once or twice a month. With the bypass, that stuff is off limits... sometimes forever. Forever is a long time not to have a Twinkie. There are a lot more complications of the bypass, as well, food wise. I've read it's a bit of a crap shoot as to what foods people will tolerate and what foods people won't. That's true for all these bariatric surgeries, but none more so than bypass.

After very little deliberation, Amanda and I decided to say no to both the lap-band and the bypass. The biggest factor for both of us was the continued maintenance and potential for reversal with the lap-band and the complications with sugar and carbs with the bypass. That left the procedure we had done, gastric sleeve.

The sleeve is an option, like the bypass, that isn't reversible, but it's a much simpler operation and tends to have fewer complications. My father liked to say the sleeve surgery doesn't change how your anatomy works; it just changes the size of your stomach. With the sleeve, somewhere around 70 to 85% of your stomach is cut away and then removed completely. What's left is the tube connecting your esophagus to your intestines, which is still stomach, just much smaller.

The sleeve has the added benefit of removing a portion of the stomach that almost entirely includes a part known as the gastric fundus. The gastric fundus produces ghrelin, a hormone that, in very simplistic terms, tells the brain it's time to eat. A lot of the urges overweight people feel to binge on food or to have things they shouldn't can be attributed, at least in part, to ghrelin. Ghrelin also helps to suppress the feeling of being satisfied once someone has eaten enough to feel full. Ghrelin is produced elsewhere in the body as well, but the gastric fundus is, by far, the largest source.

With it removed, the levels of Ghrelin in the body go way down, and a lot of those urges are greatly reduced. My father experienced this with his surgery. He described it to us by saying he just didn't need food anymore. Sure, he said, he felt hungry when his stomach was empty, and he still had cravings for the foods he liked from time to time, but he didn't feel any compulsion to eat or feel like he was being deprived if he didn't get to eat things he liked.

That sounded good to Amanda and me. I remember my life revolving around food. I would eat a meal and then immediately start thinking about and looking forward to my next meal. I would daydream about what I was going to eat. I lived to eat. Dad ate to live. Of course, he still enjoyed eating after his surgery. Food does taste good, after all, but he told us it wasn't really something he thought much about anymore.

After hearing that, and after talking to the doctor, our minds were made up. We confirmed with the surgeon that we both wanted gastric sleeve, or sleeve gastrectomy. With that choice made, we were on our way. We didn't know just how bumpy the road would be.

Chapter 13

Honestly, I'm Not Crazy

The psych exam was crazy (Ha ha). We both made an appointment to see the psychologist, and Amanda had the dubious honor of going first. Separated by about two weeks, I was able to learn just how crazy it would be before I stepped foot in the office. There were two visits for each of us. The first visit had us filling out several tests, and the second had us talking to a real live psychologist to go over the test results. My father told us a bit about his experience but was lacking in the details.

The night after Amanda finished her test, she told me all about it in no uncertain terms. "Oh, it was so stupid," she said. "The questions were dumb, and they asked the same ones over and over again." She told me, "It was just like that crazy test I took to work at the home improvement place, except way longer and with even weirder questions."

"Like what?" I asked. I was genuinely curious, but I also like to antagonize her just a little.

"Ok," she said. "Do you ever feel like someone else is controlling your thoughts?"

"Only after I got married."

"Har har." She chuckled. "Or how about this? True or false, as a girl, I have often wished that I was a boy."

"You answered no, I hope."

She rolled her eyes. "Well, yes, I answered no. But the questions were crazy, just like that, and there were hundreds. I answered one about liking to torment animals. Of course, I said yes to that one," she smiled.

I looked at her with a raised eyebrow. "Seriously?"

"Well, yeah… I mean… I torment our girls all the time."

I should interject here and mention we have two dogs. Since we can't have kids (yet), the dogs have filled that space in our lives and are almost like our children. I'm sure lots of folks can relate to that. We have a Blue Tick Hound Dog, named Shiloh, and a Belgian Malinois, named Mavis. We love them both to pieces, and they are spoiled beyond measure.

That said, my wife comes from a long line of teasers and tormenters. My father-in-law is a wonderful man… I have never known a more gentile, kind, and humble person in all my life, but he loves to tease folks and just be a general pain in the neck for the fun of it. He's the kind of guy who will tell stories until he's blue in the face, and you never quite know what's true and what's not. He'll be the kind of grandfather that tells his grandchildren false facts about everyday things that they'll believe until they're well into their teens. Something like, "There's a tube connecting your bellybutton to your butt, and if you pick at your bellybutton too much, the tube will break, and your butt will fall off!"

Amanda got a lot of that blood from him, and she constantly picks on everyone she loves… including me and the dogs. For me, it includes things like tickling, playing with my ears (which I hate), and just being a pain in the ass. "Hey honey, could you give me a hand?" *clap* *clap* *clap*. That kind of thing. For the dogs, it's messing with ears, tickling their paws, giving them big gnarly hugs, booping their noses, and other small torments that mildly annoy them but come from a place of love.

In her innocence, she interpreted the question about tormenting animals to mean the fun, clean, loving kind of torment. What the test meant was the evil, rotten, painful kind of torment. When I pointed that out, her face fell. She said, "Oh no! That's not what I meant. I totally thought they meant the fun kind. I didn't even think... but yeah... that makes sense. Damn. They're gonna think I'm crazy."

I had to laugh. I already knew she was crazy.

Even after talking to Amanda, I vastly underestimated the tests. I think there were five total, but it's all such a blur to me now that I don't remember. The first two were very quick and simple with simple questions and obvious answers. The answers were all either multiple choice, true and false, or scalar going from 1 to 5 or 1 to 10. I breezed through those two no sweat. I figured I'd have this thing done in record time.

Then I looked at the third test. Yeah, ok. No problem. It's only about 280 questions. The third test asked me to rate how much I agree with the written statement. Do I strongly agree, somewhat agree, unsure, somewhat disagree, or strongly disagree? I was supposed to agree or disagree with things like, "I really need a drink to feel relaxed," or "I'm at my best when I'm following a leader." By the end, I felt a bit tired and my hand was a little sore, but I thought I'd nailed it down ok and should be just about done. I mean, a test with almost 300 questions had to be the biggest one they had.

Nope. Meet the MMPI-2. MMPI stands for the Minnesota Multiphasic Personality Inventory test. The MMPI was my fourth test, and it was a 567-question true/false monster that ate up my afternoon like a fat kid eats a Little Debbie snack cake. This test was the one Amanda bemoaned when I talked to her about it.

This was the one where she liked to torment animals.

The questions ranged from simple, obvious, normal questions like, "I have a good appetite," or "My father was a good man," to weird, personal, and deep questions like, "Evil spirits possess me at times," and "My soul sometimes leaves my body." Throughout it all, I would mark true or false. I constantly checked my answer sheet against the test question numbers to be sure I didn't mistakenly miss a question and start answering the wrong ones in the wrong order. I wanted to make sure I didn't come across as a serial killer or used car salesman. Though, I guess, they could be fat and need surgery too.

I found myself needing to get up and stretch several times. The psychologist's office was a small home that had been converted into a doctor's office, and I took my test in one of the back bedrooms. Unfortunately, it was decorated like a small home as well. While I could appreciate the quaint old folks home aesthetic, it wasn't particularly well-suited for sitting and taking a test for hours at a time. I sat at an old writing desk with the kind of ancient wooden chair that creaked every time I shifted. It had just the faintest hint of upholstered padding for my rump to sit on, and the arms were far too close together to fit a fat guy comfortably. It seemed clear from the clientele that the lion's share of the business in this office came from bariatric patients, so clearly the decorator hadn't gotten the memo.

With a test that long, I started to question my ability to answer accurately. A lot of the questions were ambiguous and open to interpretation. "I have not lived the right kind of life." How do you answer that? Well, I mean... I'm reasonably successful and I've never murdered anyone so that's good... right? There was that time I peed in the pool, though, and I really enjoy killing bad guys in computer games. They're bad, though. And it's a game. Just a game. It's ok. I'm not a bad person. The pool was only that one time. Two times. I'll mark true. Wait, no, it said I have NOT lived the right kind of life. That should be false, I think.

It was inevitable that, eventually, I would incorrectly mark a question. Since the test was over 500 questions long, however, there was no way I could go back over and verify my answer to every one. The best I could do was make sure I marked every answer on the sheet and hope for the best. I was so happy to be done that I felt like it didn't matter if I thought I was the Queen of England; at least it was over.

The last test was laughable compared to the previous two I had taken. It was less than a single sheet long, probably around 50-60 questions. I breezed through and was oh-so-happy to be out of that chair and back into the real world where I belonged. I took my answers up to the front desk, in the living room, and rang the little bell so the receptionist could come out of her office, the kitchen, and take my answers away to be verified.

It wasn't long after that Amanda had her appointment with the psychologist to go over her results. I was shocked to discover the interview was to be done via computer with a psychologist on the other side of the country. Apparently, smell isn't a factor in determining if someone is crazy. After her interview, Amanda quickly pointed out to me, "See, look! I'm not crazy. The doctors had me tested." They gave her the all-clear for surgery, and one more hurdle was passed.

My turn came soon after. Just as before, they shuffled me off into a back bedroom, though it was a different one this time. On the little writing desk, in front of the requisite low-padding small-butted chair, was a laptop. The receptionist sat me down and dialed the psychologist using the computer. When the psychologist came up, she seemed like a nice enough lady. It was very strange having an interview with a doctor via the computer, but it didn't seem to cause any problems.

I tried to be very careful and not act too formal or too informal. I made sure to answer the questions clearly and not go into too much detail. I've watched cop shows. I know not to talk too much. That's how they get you. She asked about my family life. She wanted to know if I was happy. She asked about the role that food and eating played in my life and how I dealt with stress as it relates to food. She talked about my answers to a couple of the questions and just wanted clarification. It was a little nerve-wracking but, overall, very pleasant. I liked her.

Toward the end, she said, "Before we finish, I need to ask you about a couple of the questions you answered on the tests, ok?"

Ok, I thought, here it comes. Here comes the part where I'm a bad person who doesn't deserve to be thin.

"It shows you marked true to the question: I've had a traumatic experience in my childhood that affects my life," she said. "Can you talk more about that?"

I was a bit taken aback. "I did?" I sputtered. "I don't remember answering true to that question. I remember the question, but in my mind, the answer is false." Would she buy that? Did she think I was lying? I'm not lying, am I? I had a nice childhood… what could possibly have happened that I don't know about to cause me to answer true to that? I didn't mean to… no way, I must've…

"Oh, ok," she said.

I smiled a smile that said, 'Oh, thank God. Thank you for not pressing the issue. Can I go home now?'

"And, one more… Let's see… oh, yes. You said true when asked: I sometimes feel like someone else is controlling my thoughts."

"Well, only since I've been married." Ha! Ha ha. Ha… ha… heh… uh…

What I said out loud was, "Oh, no. I must've answered that one wrong too. Just like before, I remember the question and feel like I answered it as false."

"Ok." She looked down at her report. "I don't see anything else. Some questions we need to ask you about if you answer a certain way, and those two were the only red flags I had. After talking to you today, I don't see any psychological reason you're not a good candidate for surgery. Do you have any questions?"

I didn't.

"Good. Sounds like you have a good support group, and with your wife going through it as well, you should be able to support each other. Good luck, Ed!"

Turns out, I'm not crazy either. That's good to know.

Chapter 14

Doctors With Attitude

By the time our psych tests were through, it was getting into October. We both felt our handle on the timeline was firm. After all, according to the information we had from the bariatric center, we were only a few tests away from being ready to go. The biggest hurdle left, in our minds, was the EGD, or upper endoscopy. It's also called an esophagogastroduodenoscopy, though I think the only folks who actually use that term are doctors trying to sound smart and writers trying to up their page count. Besides the esophagogastroduodenoscopy, we each still had to do a round of blood work, as well as have an EKG performed.

The EKG, or electrocardiogram, turned out to be far simpler and quicker than I think either of us expected. Basically, it's just a test to measure the electrical signals in the heart and make sure everything is firing ok. In fact, it would be hardly worth mentioning here if it weren't for the doctor we had.

We did this test separately. When I arrived for my appointment, I was given the typical stack of paperwork to fill out, as per usual. This included a long questionnaire asking every conceivable question about my health, as per usual. I was then shuffled to a back waiting room, as per usual, and my vitals were taken by a medical assistant, as per usual. Once that was done, I expected, also as per usual, to wait another ten to fifteen minutes before anything else happened. I was pleasantly surprised when the assistant left and came back right away with a little machine on a rolling cart. She told me to take off my shirt and lie down on one of those crazy table/bed things that seem to be in every doctor's office. You know the ones with the almost see through paper that gets immediately shredded when you plop your butt down? That one.

Next, she stuck several probes on my chest and sides and told me to lie still and breathe normally. After just a few minutes, she told me I was all done and started unsticking things. I put my shirt back on, sat down in a chair, and she started rolling the machine back out to wherever it came from. On her way out, she told me the doctor would be in soon.

Ah, there's my perquisite wait for the doctor.

When he arrived, about fifteen minutes later, he asked me, almost word for word, every question on the sheet I already filled out in the waiting room. He verified I didn't have any chest pain, shortness of breath, nausea, vomiting, or a lingering desire to watch any Pauley Shore movies. Once that was done, I commented on how thorough he was being. I had no idea of the Pandora's Box I had opened.

"Yeah, well," he said, "I'm not from around here. Most of the doctors in this damn hospital don't even bother to make sure your meds don't interact, let alone check you answered your questions correctly. You have no idea how many patients I see that don't even know what operation they're getting. My God, I'd think if you were going to cut me open, I'd know what the operation was called!"

"Oh wow, that's crazy," I told him. I knew I was feeding him, but I couldn't help myself.

He went on, "Doctors around here just don't seem to care that much. They just shuffle people through the office one after the other. It's like a damn mill. And the worst? The worst are the anesthesiologists! Man, I tell you what, I don't know if I'd trust them with a bottle of valium, never mind the kind of stuff they're pumping into patients. You need to be in charge of your own healthcare around here. Make sure you know what they're doing to you."

I couldn't help myself. I had more fuel for him to burn, and I couldn't resist throwing it on the fire. I told him the true story of how Amanda's best friend was killed years ago by a different local hospital when the surgeon nicked her intestines during a hysterectomy. They didn't know it happened, and they didn't do a workup before she left the hospital to check for anything out of the ordinary. Sadly, she was gone two days later, leaving behind two children and dozens of devastated friends and family.

His eyes flashed. "Well that place is even worse if that's possible! They make me attend there two days a week, and I wouldn't be a patient at that place if I got stabbed in the lobby. That's awful. Healthcare here isn't like where I'm from. I just wanted to retire down here, but somehow, I got roped back into it. I think I'm one of the few doctors in this place that actually gives a damn."

This version, of course, is condensed and paraphrased from the actual conversation, which lasted roughly fifteen minutes. It was probably the single most entertaining doctor visit I've had in my life. As a person, I liked him. He was honest, friendly, forthcoming, and spirited to say the least. As a doctor though, I wasn't a fan. Badmouthing the entire hospital staff in front of a patient is pretty unprofessional behavior, even though I appreciated his candor. I can't complain about his work though. I got a passing grade on my EKG.

As the months wound down toward the end of the year, I found myself looking at the calendar with concern about getting everything done in our 2017 insurance period. The EGD was scarier than many of the other hurdles because it harbored a chance of even further delay should it go awry. An upper endoscopy is a procedure done to determine how your stomach and esophagus look on the inside. They look for things like hernias, ulcers, and acid reflux damage, among other things. The 'other things' is the scary part because they also look for bacteria. If they happen find some of the wrong bacteria, we would be placed on a regimen of antibiotics that would take an additional two weeks to kill it. Once it's dead, hopefully, another EGD would need to be performed and the process repeated.

If they found bacteria during either one of our procedures, it would be devastating to our timeline. Weeks were running out, and we certainly couldn't afford two more, not including the time to reschedule and perform another EGD.

The EGD needs to be completed shortly before bariatric surgery so the surgeon knows what to expect from your stomach when it comes time for them to operate. The bacteria-free certification only lasts so long before they need to re-verify. The EGD was one of the first things we scheduled, but it took almost two months before we had the procedure done and signed off.

The doctor was not what I would call… enthusiastic.

First, we had to schedule an appointment to meet him, so he could verify we each had an esophagus. Or something. In any case, they couldn't just schedule the procedure; we had to have a consultation first. We waited a month for it, and it was incredibly short.

"Ok, so we're going to put a camera down your throat and look for irregularities. It will be done in the hospital surgery center and you will be anesthetized. Any questions?"

"Um… no?"

"Ok, see you in two weeks."

One week later, each of us received a phone call informing us of the requirement to pay for the procedure before it could be performed. Apparently, doctor enthusiastic had dealt with one too many deadbeats in his illustrious career and didn't trust that he'd find three hundred dollars floating in my duodenum during the test. I wasn't thrilled to be paying for a medical procedure before I came out alive at the end, but what choice did I have?

On the day of the EGD, we arrived at the hospital happy to be getting it done but a little nervous about the whole thing. We checked in, paid the hospital what amounted to a down payment (a separate payment from the doctor, of course), and went off to what must be the most depressing surgical waiting room in all creation. It was small, cramped, dingy, and had the smallest television money can buy mounted to the wall. Most of the chairs in the room faced away from it. In the corner by the door to the pre-op center was a little window with a doorbell. We rang the bell, were told to wait, and waited.

After about an hour of waiting, the pre-op door opened, and my name was called. We both went in and informed the nurse that each of us had the procedure scheduled for today, back to back. There was some 'oooh, how sweet', 'awww, that's nice' when we told them we decided to do bariatric surgery together, and they showed us to our pre-op area. The pre-op areas were like bays in a car garage with curtains instead of doors and beds instead of lifts. I got mine first, and Amanda's would come later once they had one available.

Let me say here that I spend a lot of time in this book criticizing doctors, nurses, assistants, and office folks, and mostly, I think it's because they deserve it. There were only a few places during our journey that stood out to us as being havens of professionalism and medical dedication. The surgical center at our hospital, thankfully, was one of those places. The facilities weren't great, and the equipment was a little outdated, but the surgeons, doctors, and nurses there are some of the greatest medical professionals I've ever known. Everyone was upbeat and extremely knowledgeable.

With the exception of doctor enthusiastic, our EGD surgeon.

An hour and a half after we were brought back into pre-op, and two hours after my scheduled procedure time, doctor enthusiastic sauntered in wearing khakis and a Hawaiian shirt with palm trees and sharks on it. By that time, Amanda had her own pre-op bay and both of us were all hooked up and ready to go. For the EGD that meant shirt off, gown on, IV in, and some nifty little socks with grippy stuff on the bottom. The doctor meandered his way over to Amanda's bed, looked at her chart, looked at her, smiled wanly, and asked if she was ready. Amanda sputtered a little and said yes. The nurse told the doctor I was first. He looked at the nurse, looked toward my bay, shrugged his shoulders, and said, "Yeah. I know."

He then came over to me and performed the same routine, smile and all. I told him I was ready. He said, "Ok then, I'll see you in a few minutes." He tried to recover with a more genuine smile and threw it away at the last minute when he realized it didn't matter at this point.

Another ten minutes went by before the doctor's assistant locked down the bed and wheeled me into the tiny little room where the EGD was performed. I was hooked up to all manner of machines, flipped onto my side to face the doctor and his assistant, and asked if I was comfortable. I was, at least as much as was possible.

The assistant had me open my mouth wide, and they put a device in there to wedge it open, almost as though I were expected to bite the doctor at any moment. All the while, they were talking about the unusual number of births in the hospital that day. Oh, so that's what the little 'Rock a bye baby' jingles playing over the hospital audio system were for. I wondered what those were. They were in the middle of speculating what happened nine months ago when they put something big in my mouth. The doctor suspected the Super Bowl. Next thing I knew, I woke up with a slightly sore throat. It was a strange feeling. There was no getting sleepy, no going dark, no ramp up or ramp down... just a mild grogginess. My mind was just... off... suddenly, and then back on again. It was like I jumped through time.

The pre-op room is on the way to recovery, and as they wheeled me toward recovery, I vaguely remember giving Amanda a 'thumbs-up' gesture. I should note that I only remember it because she told me about it afterwards, and it made the memory appear in my brain. Had she not reminded me, the memory would be lost forever. For me, anesthesia is strange like that. I was clearly awake when they rolled me out, but the only part I remember is the part right after it was over and the parts she reminded me of.

According to Amanda, she remembers most of her procedure and never fell completely asleep. She said it wasn't uncomfortable or unpleasant, but she does remember seeing the video while they were doing it. For my part, I'm glad I was out.

According to our schedule, we were supposed to meet with the doctor one week later for a follow-up to get the results. Unfortunately for us, he decided that going to a conference was more important than keeping his appointments. His staff called to let us know we'd been bumped and rescheduled for his next available time slot three weeks later.

We were livid. On our next visit to the bariatric center, we threw doctor enthusiastic under the bus to anyone who would listen. It just so happened that one of the new medical assistants in the bariatric center used to work for him, and she knew the office manager over there. She said the office manager was a nice lady, and we should go ask for her by name and tell her how we're feeling.

After our bariatric visit, we did just that. The office manager for doctor enthusiastic got us squeezed in the day after he got back from his conference. We could tell she was doing her best with a bad situation. It seemed to us like the doctor did this frequently, and the office manager was used to dealing with upset patients. We left appeased.

Our follow-up was almost, but not quite, as short as the consultation.

"Ok, so you," he pointed at me, "have a hiatal hernia near where your esophagus meets your stomach." He showed us a picture. "It's not very big and shouldn't be an issue. The surgeon will probably fix it when she does the sleeve. There's no evidence of acid reflux and no other issues. You should be clear to go."

"And you," he looked at Amanda, "also have a hernia. It's a much bigger paraoesophageal hernia. I imagine the surgeon will fix this as well." He also showed us a picture of the inside of Amanda's stomach. To this day, I have no idea what I was looking at. "That will be up to her. I see very little evidence of acid reflux and no other (medical babble here). You're clear too."

We were both very relieved. We were also amazed that we each had a hernia and didn't know it. We thought it was neat that we'd be getting a hernia repair as a bonus to getting bariatric surgery. Not ever having to deal with doctor enthusiastic again was a nice prize too.

The pre-surgery blood work, our last task as far as we knew, was simple. Go in, get stuck, and go home. It wasn't until later that it would come back to haunt us.

Chapter 15

A1C Catastrophe

Sometime around September, our bariatric office told us the surgeon would not be taking patients into surgery in the latter half of December because of the holidays. That meant we had to have our surgeries done before December 15th or thereabouts. According to what we learned on our first official visit with the bariatric surgery navigator, all we had to do to get into surgery by that time was our sleep studies, the psych evaluation, blood work, an EKG, and an EGD. In addition, I was required to have signoff from a neurologist or neurosurgeon due to a brain hemorrhage I had many years ago.

In my initial bloodwork, it showed I had a high liver count; my liver enzymes were elevated. This was 'normal' for me, meaning it wasn't a surprise. An internist diagnosed me with fatty liver disease, due to my weight, a couple of years earlier. When I told the navigator this, she said they would contact my internist and get the required information to clear the liver issue before the surgery. So… no problem.

By the second week of October, as far as we knew, we had everything we needed as far as clearances for surgery. My neurosurgeon had me schedule an updated MRI and told me everything looked good after it came back. We both passed psych, we both had our EKG results and they were good, and we both had our EGD procedures done with clearance from doctor enthusiastic. We already had our sleep studies done prior to even talking about the surgery, and our final rounds of bloodwork had been done and read. I even received a call from the nutritionist informing me that my cholesterol was a little high, and I might want to talk to my GP (General Practitioner) about getting some medication for it.

All in all, we were cautiously optimistic about having our surgeries before the end of the year. Each of us imagined drinking our Thanksgiving dinner and being able to use the Thanksgiving holiday as recovery time, lessening the time we would need to take off from work. By Christmas, we envisioned, we would be almost back to eating things like turkey and mashed potatoes and gravy. Our spirits were high, and we actually looked forward to our next visit with the nutritionist, scheduled for about a week before Halloween. We hadn't been following the diet, but what did it matter? They were going to put us on a pre-op diet and didn't have any restrictions on weight gain. At least, not that we'd broken. We managed to keep our weight right at the same level it always was, while eating all the things we loved and even splurging a little, since we knew it was our last chance.

Two weeks before Halloween, I received a phone call from the bariatric center. It was brief. They simply told me I had a "couple of doctor's orders to pick up." There was no explanation, just the fact that I needed to pick them up. I felt confused by this. What did they mean, a couple of doctor's orders? Wouldn't that mean I have a couple more tests to do? I don't have any more; we've done them all.

But, apparently, we hadn't. My new doctor's orders were for a liver ultrasound to confirm my liver enzymes were, in fact, fatty liver. I also had an order for a chest x-ray. My wife received a new order for a liver ultrasound as well. It seems her liver enzymes came back high on her last round of bloodwork too. We were upset, but what could we do? At least both of those procedures could be done by the same facility and reasonably quickly. We each made our appointments.

I fretted for almost a week over the chest x-ray. The nutritionist's office didn't say what it was for, and all I could do was wonder, "What could've possibly come back in my bloodwork that would need an x-ray to diagnose?" Of course, I looked it up online, which was a mistake. By the end of that week, I was almost sure I had cancer of some kind. We each had our procedures done before the nutritionist visit, but the results would take a few more days to come back.

We met with the nutritionist together this time. Seems the office wasn't very consistent even when it came to their own rules. She chastised us mightily for not sticking to the diet. We lied, at least a little, in our food logs and made them seem far healthier than reality, but we didn't lie hard enough. The whole visit was about mistakes we were making in our food choices and had nothing to do with the surgery or any of the orders we had received a week earlier.

Finally, at the end of the visit, Amanda asked about the bloodwork.

"Oh, ok. We can go over that if you want. Edwin, I'll look at yours first."

"Ok," I said, bracing myself. The news I received was nothing like what I expected.

"Ok, so let's see... normal... normal... normal... a little high... normal... your cholesterol is high, but we talked about that, right?"

"Yes, on the phone," I said, still bracing. I couldn't hold out any longer. "Why did they want me to have a chest x-ray?"

"Oh, that's a standard pre-surgical test. Everyone gets that," the nutritionist said matter-of-factly.

"Well... I didn't get an order for that," Amanda chimed in. "Do I need one?"

"Oh, yes. If you don't have one. They didn't give you one?"

We shot a look at each other across the table that was shocked, amused, and angry all at once.

"No," Amanda said, flatly.

"Ok, well we'll get you one. I'll talk to the navigator. Everyone needs a chest x-ray; it's just a standard thing we do for all surgical patients."

Nobody ever told us that. I was all set to be angry about it until the nutritionist dropped the next bomb on my head. She didn't even realize she was doing it until it exploded in her face.

"Ok, so let's see, what else... normal... normal... oh, your A1C is 8.8, that's far too high. The surgeon won't do the surgery unless it's 7 or lower. Normal... normal..."

"Wait, what?!" I exclaimed. "Did you just say the surgeon won't do the surgery unless my A1C is less than 7?" I couldn't believe it. In her tiny little voice, with no pomp or circumstance, the nutritionist had just curb stomped my chances of having the surgery by the end of the year.

"Yep," she said. "That's her rule. So, you'll need to get that down."

"How?" I asked. "How can I possibly get my A1C, which is a six-month rolling average, down from 8.8 to under 7 in one month? Is that even possible?" I was on the verge of shouting.

"Uh..." she blinked. She didn't know how to deal with my sudden flare of indignation. If we'd been in a physical fight, she would've been rocking back on her heels. "I... I don't know. It... it could be."

"Nobody ever told me my A1C had to be below 7. That was never a requirement, as far as I knew," I continued, barking. "I know I wasn't following the diet like I should've been, but had I known about this, it would've been a different story. I need to have this surgery before the end of the year or it's going to cost me another three thousand dollars because of my insurance. Do you understand that?"

She said that she did, and she told me there was nothing she could do. She finished my blood work report and went on to Amanda's. Luckily for us, Amanda's report had no such bombshell. By the time our visit with the nutritionist was over, I was silently fuming, and Amanda looked a bit shell-shocked. Our best laid plans came unraveled, just like that.

The nutritionist escorted us over to the navigator afterwards. My mood had not improved. Before the nutritionist left the navigator's office, I confronted her again. This time, the navigator got to hear it. "I'm extremely disappointed about this. My wife and I planned on going through this together. I was never told about the A1C requirement, and now it means I almost certainly won't be able to have the surgery before the end of the year. That means we're no longer having it together, and I may not have it at all. Do you understand that? I can't afford another three thousand dollars. Had I known about the A1C requirement, I wouldn't have been treating the last few months like a dying man's last meal, knowing I won't be able to eat my favorite things ever again after surgery."

The nutritionist stammered, "I... I'm sorry." She looked on the verge of tears.

The navigator sat in her chair, wide-eyed and gape-mouthed. I turned and sat in one of her chairs, and Amanda did the same. The nutritionist retreated down the hallway.

"So, I have to get my A1C down to below 7?" I asked the navigator, hoping there was an escape clause of some kind.

"Yes, I'm sorry. That's not our rule. It's the surgeon's rule. She doesn't feel comfortable operating on anyone with an A1C higher than that," the navigator responded. I could tell she was gearing up for a struggle, but I was all struggled out.

"Do you think it's possible to lower my A1C by 1.8 points in a month?"

"I don't know. I suppose it might be. Either way, you need to do your best, don't you? Stick to the diet, and we can do another round of bloodwork to see where you are after a month," she said.

"And if I can get it down?" I asked, hopeful but tired.

"Well, I think if you get it down by early December, we should definitely be able to get both you and Amanda in by the first or second week of January," she smiled.

Again, I patiently explained our insurance situation and let her know that, under no circumstances, should this delay Amanda's surgery. By this time, my emotional pot had boiled over, and all I was left with was a lingering headache and a desire to be away from the bariatric office. I thought maybe I could talk to the doctor's nurse at some point, once I had prepared my arguments, and get some leniency or see if they would make an exception for me. I felt like it was the only hope I had left.

The navigator printed up Amanda's order for a chest x-ray and sent us on our way, assuring us once again that, other than my A1C and Amanda's chest x-ray, we should be good to go on the surgery. They were going to submit prior authorizations for both of us to our insurance company so that insurance would be ready. She told us to have a nice day.

Roughly four days after our bombshell visit with the nutritionist, I received a call from the surgeon's nurse at the bariatric center.

Honestly, I'm not sure what she even did for that office. She didn't attend during either of our surgeries, and we almost never saw her in the office until about a week before Amanda's surgery when we attended her pre-op 'class.' She teaches classes and deals with medication issues, mostly, I think, and sort of acts like a liaison between the surgeon and the bariatric center nutritionists. She called to give me an update on my x-ray and see how things were going.

"Edwin, hi! So, I'm calling because I wanted to let you know your x-ray came back clear, no issues there. What do you have left? Let's see... I don't have all the paperwork in front of me. Did you ever get your liver ultrasound done?"

"Yes."

"Ok, because I don't have it. Can you call the imaging center and see if they'll transfer it over to us? I'll give you my fax number." She recited it.

I wrote it down. I braced myself for bad news and asked the question I'd been wondering for days. "So, when I talked to the nutritionist, she said my A1C was too high for surgery."

"Yeah," she said in a way that was pleasantly patronizing. "Surgeon's requirements are under 7. Yours, as of your last bloodwork... when was that?" she asked.

"October 9th," I replied.

"Right. It was 8.8, which is way up there. Unfortunately, the surgeon is pretty strict about this sort of thing, so we'll need you to get that down."

I stiffened a little. "So there's no way to make an exception? Even if, say, in a month, I get tested and I'm down over a full point to 7.7 or something?"

"No Edwin, I'm sorry. It's for your safety. I know you don't like to hear this, but everything we do we do for your health. If your A1C is too high, it can cause complications."

I spent the better part of the next 30 minutes trying to rationalize why I should be able to have the surgery before the end of the year. I told her I would sign a waiver. No good. I told her I wasn't informed of the requirement. She told me that she could neither confirm nor deny I was telling the truth, but all patients are supposed to be informed. It didn't matter anyway; safety was safety. I pleaded with her, telling her I wouldn't be able to have the surgery if I couldn't get it done this year. It didn't faze her; she simply told me we would need to re-evaluate things once I got my numbers below 7. She then told me that, due to my attitude and the way I was carrying on about it, maybe I wasn't ready for the surgery after all.

Toward the end of the conversation, I shifted gears and began pleading on behalf of Amanda. I told the nurse that at least Amanda needed to get it done before the end of the year because we wanted to have a baby, and the weight loss would help her conceive. The nurse immediately made me promise not to attempt to get Amanda pregnant within a year of her surgery and even went so far as threatening to make me sign a document saying as much. She briefly went over Amanda's paperwork and told me there was a good chance that Amanda could be seen before the end of the year, but there were no guarantees.

Looking back, I think I can say with some certainty that the end of that phone conversation was the lowest point of my entire 2017. I threw every argument, every emotion, every piece of ammunition at that nurse, and she didn't budge. I slumped into my chair at the end, completely defeated, hoping they would take pity on us and allow Amanda to have her surgery before the surgeon stopped for the holidays. The focus now was on her and making sure she took care of any remaining tasks.

The only thing I could do for myself was to lower my A1C. I read somewhere on the internet that donating blood can quickly lower your A1C, so hopefully, I saved a life that month. We had a gigantic bowl of candy left over from Halloween, which I didn't touch at all after Halloween, even though my father would grab a handful and happily munch on it every time he came over. We already had food, good food, planned for our last few weeks of eating like normal people. Most of it went in the garbage.

From Halloween until my pre-op diet, I followed the low carb diet like it was my new religion. The only exception was Halloween. Amanda and I have a tradition of ordering a pizza and watching "*It's the Great Pumpkin, Charlie Brown,*" while trick or treaters visit, so we went to the store and found the thinnest crust pizza they had. I also had two fun-sized candy bars. Subway salads became my new go-to meal, and we each fired up Pinterest again in an effort to de-carb our lives. Amanda followed the diet, as well, because it was just easier for each of us to have the same meals. Over the course of the next month, I lost 15 lbs. I hoped it would be enough.

Chapter 16

In the Nick of Time

During the afternoon of November 16th, Amanda received a call from the bariatric center. They were ready to schedule her for surgery. They asked if she would be ok with having her surgery on the 28th of November, and she immediately said yes. Excited and nervous, she called me as soon as she was off the phone with them. I was stunned. I can't exactly describe the precise mixture of emotions I felt at that moment, but whatever the concoction was, it was enough to leave me speechless and surprisingly unsure.

You might wonder why I would be unsure, and so did I. I couldn't believe that part of my brain was screaming, "Don't! It's too soon! Not enough time! Not fair!" It seems fear, and even jealousy, found their way into my thoughts. With my own surgery being denied for 2017, I had a distinct feeling of envy that I just couldn't shake. A few seconds into the phone call though, logic took over, and I told her the truth of it: It was fantastic news. No more waiting, no more wondering, no more hoops, and no more tests!

That, unfortunately, turned out to be wrong. They had a whole slew of new tasks for Amanda to complete. She needed a new CPAP compliance report to make sure she was actually using the sleep apnea machine. She needed to get pre- and post-op chewable vitamins, since you can't swallow a vitamin whole after surgery. She needed new appointments with the office nurse and the surgeon.

The nurse's appointment was a class that all pre-op surgery patients were required to attend. It was scheduled on the same day as her appointment with the surgeon, and I decided to tag along. I thought maybe they would give me credit for the class, so I wouldn't need to take it when my time came. It also gave me a shot in the dark chance at talking to the surgeon, personally, about my own situation. I didn't hold out much hope, but it was worth a shot.

The class attendance was small, only about four people, including me. I wasn't registered officially for the class, so they told me I wasn't going to get credit for attending. Miffed, I waited with Amanda for the nurse to arrive and start the class. She led us all down to another, unused, waiting room, and handed out books to everyone but me. The class went over what the pre-op and post-op diet requirements were, how to take care of your incisions, how the surgery was likely to go, and how to handle recovery.

We already knew the pre-op requirements, but she went over them again. For two weeks prior to surgery, we would be on a liquid diet apart from one meal per day. That meal was to be four to six ounces of lean protein with two to three ounces of vegetables or other non-carb food. The nurse didn't explain why; she rarely explained the why of anything, but research online provided an answer for the pre-op diet. Turns out, your liver is pretty much completely in the way while the surgeon is doing her thing. To make it more manageable, the diet has the effect of shrinking your liver size. Apparently, your liver likes to get fatty, I know mine does, and it's just about the first place fat comes off when you lose weight. Sticking to a pre-op diet does your surgeon a favor by making dealing with your liver far easier.

For three weeks after the surgery, we would live on nothing but fluid while our stomachs healed. Protein shakes and water, for the most part. Sugar and caffeine free drinks were ok, as was sugar free Jell-O and sugar free popsicles.

During those three weeks, we would be required to log every sip we took in a journal. We had to get 70 grams of protein every day and at least 64 ounces of clear liquid. Immediately following the surgery, we would be given ice chips to suck on and melt in our mouth, NOT to swallow. The nurse encouraged us to practice melting ice in our mouths in the weeks leading up to surgery. We would not be cleared to swallow anything after the surgery until they verified everything was leak free the following morning.

The nurse informed us we would receive instructions on how to eat after the three-week period during our next class, one week after surgery.

The surgery would be done laparoscopically, which means they only make four or five small incisions and insert tools inside to do the surgery using cameras. We thought that was neat and were glad to know we weren't going to have a huge scar. We were all told we might have a drain installed after surgery to help with removing excess air. Air? Turns out, they pump your abdomen full of CO_2, so they have more room to work with. They try to drain as much as they can, but air is tricksy and likes to find places to hide, so they might require a drain to get more of it out afterwards. If so, we would be shown how to care for it. The incision points would be sewn inside with dissolving sutures and then covered with surgical glue on the outside. We were to leave the surgical glue alone. It would fall off eventually when it got tired of our shit.

After the class, Amanda and I went back into the bariatric center waiting room and stuck around until her appointment with the surgeon. When it finally came, we went through the standard wait, underling, wait, vitals, wait routine. Finally, the surgeon came in and did a brief checkup on Amanda. They went over the type of surgery, possible complications (up to and including death), and, at the end, she asked if Amanda had any questions. Amanda did not. The surgeon said, "Great! Then I'll see you again on the 28th."

Backtracking here for a moment, I should note that, by this time, it was almost three weeks since I'd been strictly on the low carb diet. Just a few days earlier, I'd talked to the nutritionist and requested another blood test to check my A1C. The A1C came back at 7.7. I had dropped an entire point in three weeks, but not enough to bring me below the 7.0 threshold.

As the surgeon turned to leave, I knew this was my chance; it was now or never. I hated to do this during Amanda's appointment, but I didn't have a choice. Amanda knew it was coming. I had her permission, but I had to be careful. I didn't want to screw this up.

"Doc, I have a quick question," I said.

"Sure, go ahead," she turned and raised an eyebrow.

"I was wondering… a month ago, my A1C came back as 8.8. They told me that's too high to have the surgery. Can you tell me why the A1C makes a difference?" I tried to be matter-of-fact and unemotional.

"Sure," she said. "High blood sugar levels have many negative effects on the body, and one of those is recovery. It takes your body longer to heal if you have uncontrolled high blood sugar, so we ask that patients keep it below 7 for their own safety and to expedite the healing process as much as possible."

"Oh, ok," I looked at her with just a hint of an upturned eyebrow myself. "I've dropped my A1C to 7.7 in the last three weeks by sticking to the diet. My average blood glucose has been between 90 and 110 during that time. Since my actual blood sugar is so low, and I've dropped my A1C by so much, would it be possible to make an exception for me, so I could have the surgery before the end of the year?"

It was out. I'd made my pitch. This was the last chance I had. My face didn't flinch, but every synapse in my brain was puckered.

"I don't think that would be a problem. Tell you what, we'll go ahead and schedule you for this year and take another look right before the surgery date. So long as you stay below where you are now, 7.7, I should be able to do it. I reserve the right to cancel, though, if I see anything in your food log I don't like." There was just a hint of a smile playing on her lips. "Just don't tell anyone I made an exception."

My heart leapt into my throat. "No problem, Doc. I'll be good for sure."

"Ok then, I'll tell the navigator to get you scheduled. Amanda, I'll see you in a few days."

I was overjoyed. Cloud 9, all the way. I floated over to the navigator room, with Amanda on my heels. The navigator was glad to hear the doctor gave me a pass. I think she was mostly glad I wasn't pissed off anymore. She looked through the doctor's schedule and found a date: December 14th. I told her I would definitely take it.

"You still need to take the pre-op class, right?" she asked.

"Well, technically, yes. I was there this morning with Amanda though." I rolled my eyes, just slightly.

"Let's see if we can make that count for you." She dialed the office nurse.

"Hi, I'm with Edwin. We just got him scheduled for surgery. He said he was in the class with you this morning... uh huh... ok. Hold on. Edwin, do you feel like you retained enough of the class to be ok with it or would you like to go through it again?"

"Oh, I got it. No problem," I said quickly.

"Yeah, he's got it. Ok, great. Thanks." She hung up.

"Ok, that's done. Uh, let's see... did you ever get your ultrasound."

Dammit, I thought. With all the stuff going around, I completely forgot to call them, and I told her as much.

"Oh, no problem, just a sec." She dialed the imaging center, asked for the ultrasound, gave them her fax number and said, "Done. What's next... Oh! Look. I have a cancellation on the 7th. Would you like to go then?"

Wow, this was happening fast. In my mind, I was quickly trying to calculate if the 7th would put me in the two-week pre-op diet during Thanksgiving. Sure, it did. Hell, it put me in the pre-op diet NOW. I didn't really want that, but how could I bitch and moan about not getting it done this year and then turn around and say no when given an earlier date?

"Uh... yea... yeah. Yeah, that would be fine," I stammered. I looked over at Amanda. Her eyes were glowing, and she was smiling. We were scheduled within ten days of each other, and we were having it done before the end of the year.

Chapter 17

Down to the Wire

I made an appointment with my GP just to make sure all my meds were properly filled before my surgery. The bariatric center didn't seem to require my GP to know what was going on, but the last thing I needed was to run out of meds during my recovery. Getting appointments with our GP can take a few days, even up to a week, so I called well before my surgery date. They got me an appointment, and I was all set.

The day of my appointment, a week to the day before Amanda's surgery and during the week of Thanksgiving, the bariatric center called Amanda and said her last task was getting approval from her GP, which is the same doctor as mine. This was on a Tuesday, and her surgery was scheduled for the following Tuesday. Thanksgiving was Thursday, and the GP's office was closed Thursday and Friday. Neither of us could believe it. Not once had they told us we needed anything from our GP doctor, and now, suddenly, one week before Amanda's surgery, we needed his sign-off. As I said, getting in to see him was notoriously difficult sometimes, let alone during the holidays. To say we were worried would be understating it.

Amanda called and called that day, trying to get an appointment. She was put on hold, disconnected, put on hold again, and finally talked to the receptionist. The earliest appointment they had available was at 8:15 am on Monday, the day before her surgery. When she told me, I asked her to switch appointments with me. After all, I already had my appointment scheduled. If we swapped, she would have more time to deal with anything that came up. For my part, I had plenty of time before my procedure, so if something came up, I'd be able to deal with it.

We asked the doctor's office if we could switch, and they refused. They gave us some line about other patients being on a waiting list and that they would be slotted in my spot first if I cancelled. I told them I wasn't cancelling, just having my wife take my spot. They told me that means I would need to cancel. Frustrated, I hung up. It seemed there was no way to push her appointment up, at least not over the phone. I hoped I would be able to sweet talk the doctor into seeing her sooner during my appointment.

When I saw him, I opined to the doctor how frustrated I was. He told me he was shocked the bariatric center only just told us about the requirement for a GP to sign off. He almost acted hurt or insulted that they didn't seem to care about him. He asked about me, and I told him my surgery was scheduled for the 7th of December, about a week and a half after Amanda's.

"Well, you're here," he said, "might as well give you a pre-surgery examination, so it's out of the way. It looks like you're missing some lab and test work that I need to sign off on, so you'll need to get those results from the bariatric center and bring them by sometime."

I was used to that. For some reason, even though all the doctors and offices were in the same hospital network, many of them either didn't realize the records were shared or didn't know how to access them. For the doctors, it was far simpler to ask the patient to get a paper copy and bring them along.

He had me hop up on that dumb little table/bed thing and start coughing and breathing. I was told to lie back, and he rubbed several different spots on my body, checking for whatever it is that swells when things aren't going right. I sat back up and he made me follow his pen with my eyes, checked that I knew how to grip his finger, and looked in my ears to make sure my hamster was still running.

"Ok, stand up over here. Good, now take down your pants," he said in the very casual way that, it seems, doctors must learn in doctor school.

I took them down.

"Um... underwear too. Yeah. I need to check... mumble bumble..." he trailed off, like what he wanted to check was unspeakable.

I took my underwear down as well, and now we were both in that awkward place that only exists between a male doctor and his male patient. The awkwardness didn't improve when he grabbed my junk. I thought to myself, "Oh, well. Here we are now. This is happening." It was over as soon as it began, and I could tell the doctor was glad it was done. He did a good job of staying professional about it, but there was no mistaking the hint of relief in his face. I had no idea what a doctor could possibly check by squeezing my dangly bits, but it must've been important.

After telling me everything looked good, medically, he refilled my meds and told me I was good to go so long as I got him the paperwork he needed. I asked him if there was anything he could do about Amanda's appointment time.

"No, I'm sorry. The front office makes the appointments, and if there isn't anything available, there's nothing I can do. 8:15 Monday should give us plenty of time to get her approved for surgery on Tuesday though. I wouldn't worry too much."

I wasn't entirely sure I believed that, but what could we do? I found myself capitulating far more than I liked. There was no other option.

Amanda's appointment day came. While I went to work, she went to the doctor's office to get clearance from the GP. I was worried but tried to rationalize it away. After all, what could the doctor possibly find that would block Amanda from having the surgery? The bariatric center already cleared her on their end and so had the hospital. The GP wasn't going to have a problem with anything already cleared by the actual surgeon.

Except that he did. Of course, he did. The day before Amanda's surgery, our GP found a problem.

Amanda's liver ultrasound from a week or so earlier had come back and showed that her spleen was just a bit enlarged. The report about it was plain as day, so the surgeon and hospital knew. Amanda and I knew as well. We weren't worried in the slightest because, we figured, if the surgeon doesn't care and the hospital doesn't care… why should we? Turns out, our GP cared. Even though it could've easily been a shadow or other imaging artifact, the GP felt it was serious enough to warrant a CT scan, "Just to make sure."

Mortified, Amanda reiterated our situation to him. She told him her surgery was scheduled for the next day, and that we'd been working on this for months. She asked him how she could ever make her surgery time if she needed a CT scan, which takes days to schedule and then days more to review. She asked him why he cared if the surgeon and hospital didn't. Finally, in desperation, she turned on the water works.

It was very effective.

The GP didn't drop his requirement for a CT scan, but he did set up an order for a CT scan to be done at the hospital stat. I always thought stat was one of those dumb things you hear in medical movies and TV shows that real professionals don't say… like when folks on CSI or NCIS tell some tech nerd to enhance a video. "Enhance! Enhance! Enhance! See? There, flip the image. You can clearly see the writing on the back of that guy's hand by viewing the reflection in the window of the shop behind him. Case solved!"

Stat is a real thing. I read on the Googles that stat comes from the Latin word statum, meaning 'immediately.' That was appropriate, because they got Amanda into her CT scan at the hospital almost immediately. When she went to register, they even gave her a special card that allowed her to cut in front of the line. The GP had assured her that he would have the results by the end of the day and, if all was well, she would have her clearance.

It was a rough day for both of us. Amanda spent her time in the hospital getting poked, prodded, and scanned and then waiting the rest of the day for the results. I spent my day at work, feeling utterly useless and wishing there was some way to help. Amanda suffered the additional hardship of being forbidden from eating any real food.

The full day before surgery, we weren't allowed to eat anything and could only drink protein drinks and water. They asked us to drink as much water as possible, at least half our body weight in ounces. Presumably, this is so we didn't get dehydrated before, during, and immediately after the surgery. It seems like it would've been rough on its own, but I can't imagine what it was like for Amanda with the added stress of the CT scan.

It took until the end of the day to hear back. The GP doesn't view lab and test results until the end of the day, a fact the receptionist made abundantly clear to both Amanda and the bariatric center nurse whenever they called to get the results. Finally, it turns out, the test was clear. Whatever it was that showed up on the ultrasound did not show up in the CT scan. Amanda's insides were in the right places and of the right proportions. We had finally cleared the last possible hurdle for her surgery, and she was to be at the hospital the next day around noon.

Chapter 18

Amanda Goes First

We arrived around 11:30 am, just to make sure we had plenty of time. Amanda packed a big overnight bag full of all kinds of things like pajamas, phone chargers, extra socks, and even a book. She never used most of it. After signing in at the front desk, this time without stat, we sat in the waiting area and watched the comings and goings of people. I found myself wondering if any of the other folks there were waiting for bariatric surgery. There were definitely a couple of candidates, which is a nice way of saying they were fat, too.

After roughly twenty minutes, Amanda's name was called, and we went back to an office in the reception area to sign in. There, after some paperwork, pleasantries, and standard disclaimers, a nice lady told us we would owe the hospital somewhere around $1800 and would that be cash or charge? I told her Amanda was near her out-of-pocket limit on our insurance, the entire reason we fought so hard to get this done before the end of the year, and I wasn't sure how much more we had to go. The check-in attendant told us she didn't know either, but we had to put something down today, or they wouldn't check us in.

Amanda and I looked at each other and shrugged. It was what it was. More capitulation because, 'What could you do?' I sighed and told the registrar we could pay $200 with a credit card. She seemed happy enough with that, and, now that the nasty business of money was out of the way, wished Amanda great success, gave her the requisite hospital arm band, and told us how to get to surgery.

A few days earlier, I had been ordered to have a CT scan done as well. My liver ultrasound came back showing something strange around my pancreas, and they wanted to be sure it was nothing before my surgery. As with my x-ray, I Googled and searched to see what I had. Cancer, of course. Must be. Since I would be taking Amanda to the hospital for her surgery, I figured the day of her surgery would be a good day for me to get my CT scan. Two birds with one stone. After Amanda's check in, I checked in for my CT scan as well. No charge. I already hit my max out-of-pocket.

They didn't care when I had my scan done. I figured I would do it while Amanda was either getting prepped or while she was in surgery, so we wandered back into the most depressing surgical waiting room in the universe, once again. We still couldn't get one of the few seats facing the television, coveted by all surgical waiting room denizens, so we just sat and pulled out our phones. There was very little to talk about. Months of waiting, stress, being seen by doctors, and being annoyed by offices had worn us out, and we knew this was the calm before the storm.

It was probably about 1:30 before they called Amanda's name. We went back and were greeted by the World's Greatest Nurse. He didn't have a T-Shirt or coffee mug saying so, but he should've. I've tried to stay away from calling people out in this book, so I tend not to give out names, but in this case, I'll make an exception. His name was Lee, and I'm damn glad he was there for us during our surgeries. We were both blessed to have him as our pre-op nurse. He made getting prepped far less stressful.

Lee led Amanda back to her pre-op stall, and I followed, carrying her bag. He went over paperwork, asked her name, double checked the procedure she wanted done, her doctor's name, and went over her medications. It was interesting to think that, should all go well, I would be doing this same routine in about a week. Lee brought Amanda her gown, drew the curtain, leaving Amanda and me alone, and asked her to change into the gown. "Nothing but gown and socks. Two pair of socks, yellow first, then brown on top of those. I'll tell you why in a minute."

She put on the gown and socks, yellow socks first, and got up on the bed. Next was the part that, I think, Amanda dreaded the most. Amanda hates being stuck by needles, to the point where she will turn white and get nauseous if she even thinks about it too much. It was time for the IV, and Lee came in with the needle. The gauge was pretty large, since it needed to push a lot of fluid. He asked Amanda which arm she wanted, and she didn't care. He looked at both of her arms and determined that her right would be more convenient for movement, but her left had a better vein. He decided to try the right arm. It was a mistake.

He poked. She winced. He rooted for the vein, trying, but not finding it. She started to tear up. Lee gave it his best shot, but, ultimately, he couldn't get it. Amanda and I tend to be hard to stick. He pulled the needle out, put a bandage on her right arm, and moved to the left. He apologized but had to get the stick done. This time, on the left arm, he got it right away.

"Damn," he said to himself, "shoulda' went with my gut. The vein on your left arm was much better. I'm sorry about that."

Amanda's face was white. She did her best to smile and nod, but I could tell she was mainly focused on not passing out.

After that, there was little more to do but wait. Lee checked her abdomen for anything that might cause a concern and verified a few other things. We chatted a little with Lee about how the two of us were going through surgery together. In fact, I told him I was scheduled to do a CT scan that very day for my own surgery, nine days later.

"Well then," he said, "you should go ahead and get that done. The doctor has at least one more surgery to go before Amanda goes back. I figure she has about another hour to wait, so you have time. If you get back here by around 3:45, just come on back. If not, check with the pre-op desk and see if Amanda's still waiting. If I don't see you then, I'll hopefully see you in about a week!"

I gave Amanda a kiss and took off for my CT scan. The radiology waiting room was smaller than the surgical one but not as depressing. I was a little stressed about the time, so I anxiously watched the clock while I waited. The minutes ticked by. I had the entire waiting room to myself, so I wondered what could possibly be taking so long. Eventually, around 3:25, someone came in and ushered me back to where the machine was.

I removed any accessories I had, belt, phone, wallet, keys. They had me lie down on a slab in front of the machine. The CT machine was large, consisting almost entirely of a gigantic ring. It was clear that the slab, with me on it, would move through the ring once the procedure started. The radiology nurse came with a needle for my IV, and he had no problem finding my vein. I was moving in and out of the ring before I knew it.

After a few cycles, the nurse announced they would now add 'contrast' via the IV. Contrast is a medical term for adding something to the blood, such as iodine, barium, or gadolinium, which causes things to show up differently during imaging scans. It helps the doctor see things better.

It also makes you feel like you just pissed yourself.

An otherworldly warming feeling passed throughout my body, starting in my groin. It took every ounce of logic and willpower I had to resist the urge to reach down there and feel if my crotch was wet. As the feeling permeated the rest of me, I realized it was the contrast and settled down. The feeling was incredibly strange, almost like I was submerged in a hot tub, but obviously without the water. It subsided after five or ten seconds, then I was finished. They unhooked me, gave me back my things, and I was free to go.

It was 3:45 on the nose. I fast walked back to surgery pre-op and rang the little receptionist door-bell. When I asked about Amanda, they told me she was still waiting to go in, but it wouldn't be long. They buzzed me back.

When I got to her stall, she was completely prepped. She even had one of those little paper shower caps and some weird kind of air bladders on her legs. I found out later they inflated and massaged the legs to promote blood flow during extended inactivity. Inactivity wasn't a problem at the moment though; everything was abuzz. It seems I had arrived right on time. There was a surgical nurse getting Amanda up out of the bed, so she could take her walk into surgery.

Our surgeon had a policy. Everyone walks into surgery. She did this because she strongly felt that bariatric surgery should be the decision of the patient, and the patient should be ultimately responsible for bringing themselves to the operating table. She wanted all her patients to feel empowered that the decision was theirs, and that they were making their own journey. That was the reason for the two pairs of socks. The outer pair, brown, were used for the walk into the operating theatre. After that, the brown pair was removed and discarded, so the clean yellow pair could be used during surgery and subsequent recovery.

By the time I reached her, Amanda was all the way up on her feet. She saw me coming and gave me a big smile.

"Hey, you just made it! Get your CT scan done?"

"Yep, all set," I replied.

"Good."

"Glad I made it back in time to see you off."

"Me too," she smiled. I could tell she was a little nervous but also ready. The nurses were waiting for us to finish before the surgical nurse took her back to the OR.

"Good luck, sweets. This is what we've been waiting for. I love you. See you in a little bit," I offered with my own smile.

"Thanks, I love you too," she leaned in and gave me short little kiss. She looked at the nurse and gave a slight nod. They were off. I watched them walk, slowly, down the hall toward the big double doors that break the pre-op area from the operating rooms. She looked back and waved. I did the same.

Now, all I could do was wait. I went and sat in the most depressing surgical waiting room in the universe, still not able to acquire a spot in front of the television. My phone was running dry, and there was nothing to do. Luckily for me, my parents arrived after just a few minutes. We'd been in communication, so they knew what was going on and where we were in the process. Amanda's parents lived about 90 minutes away, and unlike my parents, weren't retired, so they were stuck at work and couldn't make it. They would see her the next day.

The three of us waited together while the clock slowly ticked away the minutes and seconds. Generally, we just made small talk. Dad let me use his portable phone charger and bragged about how well it worked. I was impressed with it and told him so. He and Mom talked a little about his surgery and how she had to wait for him to get out. There wasn't much else to do, other than small talk and people watch, which was not what I would call fun in a surgical waiting room. Some folks weren't very happy to be there.

Eventually, around 4:45, the surgeon popped in and looked around. I waited for her to notice me and, failing that, began to wave to get her attention. When she finally caught sight of me, she smiled and walked over.

"Hi. Amanda did fine. Everything is looking good. The surgery is over, and I was able to repair her hernia as well," she stated. It was almost rehearsed. I imagine this is something she said several times a week.

"Ok, so no problems at all?" I knew the answer, but somehow felt hearing it one more time would be best.

"No, no problems at all. She's in recovery but still sleeping. She should wake up in about an hour, then you'll be able to see her."

"Ok, thanks, doc." I made sure to look her in the eye as I said it, so she knew I meant it. I did mean it.

"Of course. You folks have a good evening," again, rehearsed, but not insincere. She turned and walked out into the hall, off to wherever it is doctors go when they're done. Amanda was her last surgery that day.

Finally, after a little more than an hour, a nurse came into the waiting room and looked around. "For Amanda Zeninski?" I sighed. Everyone always pronounces our last name wrong. I ignored it, as I almost always do, and got up to go see my wife.

Chapter 19

A Husband's Duty

Amanda was in the recovery room on one of those wheeled hospital beds. Her post-op nurse was professional but a little surly. I imagined she had to be. She spent most of her time telling post-op patients to do things they don't want to do. Things like walking and blowing into an incentive spirometer. When I arrived, she had me sit next to Amanda and gave me a cup of ice with a spoon.

"Do you have her spirometer?" the nurse inquired.

"Oh, no," I replied. "It's out in her bag."

"You need it. Go get it," she grumbled.

I went and got it. The incentive spirometer was a little device made from clear and blue plastic. It had a little plunger/bobber inside and a clear hose made to look like it should be blown into. On the main housing, holding the plunger, were marks from 0 to 4000 and a little blue arrow that could be moved up and down the scale. The idea was that you would move the blue arrow to your target number and then manipulate the machine to get the plunger up to the target. It looked easy, but the trick is that you suck on it, not blow into it.

Sucking is harder than blowing, so getting the plunger up to a respectable number is deceptively hard. It's incredibly hard just after you've had three quarters of your stomach cut out and five incisions in your abdomen as a result of surgery. No matter, it was a requirement to use the machine three times every fifteen minutes at a minimum for the first week. Doing so exercises the lungs and prevents pneumonia.

When I got back with Sucky McSuckface (my name for the spirometer), Amanda was groggy and still not fully awake. Every so often, she would look at me and ask for a piece of ice to melt in her mouth. I gladly obliged. I tried talking to her a little, but she wasn't in much condition for chatting. I told her I was proud of her and that everything went well. She smiled wanly. It was clear she was in a lot of pain. She complained about it several times to the nurse and to me, but the nurse did little other than tell her that walking was the only way to get rid of it and make sure she was using the spirometer. Amanda rubbed her chest over and over… the air bubbles in there must've hurt like hell. She has an incredible tolerance for pain, and I'd never seen her like this.

I felt awful making her use the spirometer, but it was a requirement and my job to force her to use it. Each time the nurse glanced at me and then down at the spirometer, I felt a pang of guilt… like I was doing a piss poor job forcing my wife to suck on something she clearly didn't want to.

After 20 minutes or so, Amanda was awake enough to look around and understand where she was. The pain was still intense, but at least the grogginess was melting away. I could tell she was getting restless. The nurse had told her several times that walking was the only way to fix the pain. Walking would encourage the gas bubbles to move and, eventually, dissipate, and they were what was causing the discomfort. Amanda took this to heart and wanted to get up and walk as soon as possible.

Unfortunately, the nurse was a very busy lady. Once they had me back there, I became something of a babysitter. I dispensed ice, said encouraging things, offered up Sucky McSuckface every fifteen minutes, and looked generally like a lost husband was supposed to look. I wasn't about to take it upon myself to get Amanda up out of the bed. Never mind the fact that she had wires all over the place. Amanda knew I was pretty powerless, so she waited.

When the nurse returned, Amanda told her she wanted to walk. It came out, "I waa waak."

"Ok honey, that's good. Let's get you up. Mr. Amanda, why don't you come over and give her a hand. You can walk arm-in-arm around post-op." Ok! I had my marching orders. Do this. I can do that.

Amanda slowly swung her legs over the side of the bed, while the nurse started unplugging things. Some machine started beeping angrily. I think it was the leg massager. Finally, Amanda got all the way up and sighed heavily. She tried to stretch a little, but her sore stomach muscles made that a hard feat to accomplish. She groaned and started shuffling her feet out towards the hall. I fell in beside her on her left. The nurse was on her right.

The post-op room was just like the pre-op room. It had bays for all the patients, and Amanda certainly wasn't alone. Unlike the pre-op room, the bays were separated by only a curtain. The three of us, Amanda, the nurse, and I, shuffled together out into the main corridor. It was an L shaped room with bays on each side and the nurse's station in the crook of the L. Amanda's bay was at the lower right corner of the L.

As we shuffled, the nurse gave Amanda words of encouragement. I did my best to do the same without sounding like a jackass. "Hey, you're doing great!" I would say, as though I were talking to a three-year-old instead of my 30-year-old wife. She moaned; we shuffled. She groaned; we shuffled. She really was doing well, considering how recently the surgery happened, but even so, at one point, she started to lose her balance. The nurse and I steadied her. By this time, we had made it almost halfway to the top of the L, and Amanda indicated she was ready to go back.

Once back in the bed, Amanda asked for more ice. That was my job. I could do that. Feeding her ice with a spoon made me feel useful, and I was happy to do it. In the background, I could hear the nurses talking amongst themselves about a room upstairs. I mentioned it to Amanda. I couldn't wait for her to get her own room, and neither could she. Having her own room was the next step, like graduating from post-op, and it meant more freedom and privacy.

The next time I saw the nurse, I asked her about it. She told me they were just waiting for the room to be cleaned and then Amanda could go upstairs. I glanced at the clock, it was almost 7pm. My tummy grumbled. I was on my pre-op diet at this point and hadn't had a bite to eat since around 5 the previous day. I tried to decide what I was going to do for dinner… I didn't have anything at the house, so it would have to be out. I would have to cheat, but only a little. Amanda broke my thought.

"Ice."

I gave her some.

She said she wanted to move. It came out, "I waan moo. Oooh, it huurs."

"I know sweetheart. I'm sorry it hurts." I looked on, helplessly.

"Chess huurs. Bad. Uhmm," then a sigh.

We went on like this until the nurse finally arrived with the news that Amanda was ready to be moved. It was 7:30.

While they prepped her for departure, I let her know I was going to go back and see my parents. It had been over an hour and a half since I left them in the waiting room. I put Sucky down on the bed, gave Amanda a little peck on the lips, told her I loved her, and went back out to the waiting room. My parents, bless their hearts, were right where I left them.

By the time the three of us got upstairs, Amanda was walking again. I'll never forget the sight of her walking down the hallway towards us as we departed the elevator. A nurse was with her, steadying her as she walked, and Amanda's face was twisted up in agony. Each step she took squeezed fresh tears from her eyes. My mother's hand went up to her mouth and she whispered, "Oh, sweetie…" under her breath. My father smiled with compassion and recognition. He'd been there.

He walked up to Amanda. "It gets better. It gets better. This is the worst of it."

Amanda managed a smile through the tears and nodded slightly. The nurse helped her turn around and walk back to her room with the three of us behind. It was slow and a bit awkward but also short. Once back in the room, Amanda collapsed back into the bed and sighed. She complained about her chest hurting once again, and my mother, no stranger to doctors or hospitals, spoke up.

"Excuse me, nurse? Is there anything you can do? Can you get her some pain medication?" Mom doesn't tend to mince words.

"The best way to fight the pain is to walk, but... yes, we can give her something. She's already had some in post-op, but we can give her something else that should help with the pain and help her sleep."

Amanda seemed relieved to hear that. I certainly was. Thanks, Mom.

Not long after that, Mom and Dad said their goodbyes and departed. Amanda was clearly worn out and ready for whatever fitful sleep awaited her, so there was little else to do. I asked if she needed anything. She did not. I told her I loved her, was proud of her, and would see her first thing in the morning. She smiled and told me she loved me back. After a small peck on the mouth, tinted with a slight metallic taste from her medication, I left her be.

Though my day was much easier than Amanda's, I was also worn out and ready for bed... but not before I hit up Subway and got a salad. It was a cheat, no doubt. Far larger than six ounces and loaded with mayo and processed meat, it hit my tongue like a freight train of sin. I relished every bite. Our nutritionist would've had a conniption. I cared very little.

I was up bright and early the next morning to see how Amanda was doing. Better, but still in a fair bit of pain, she was mostly awake when I arrived at her room. She walked the halls a few times during the night between bouts of sleep. Her job this morning was to continue sucking on ice, walk whenever possible, use Sucky McSuckface, and stay out of the bed. To punctuate that last bit, a nurse came in soon after Amanda was out of the bed and removed all the sheets, so there was only an ugly vinyl covered mattress.

"No more laying in the bed. Doctor's orders are that you either sit in the chair or walk around after your first night," the nurse droned while removing the sheets.

That suited Amanda just fine. Walking did help in the grand scheme, of course, but it also helped in the moment. Walking diverts the attention away from the pain. With that in mind, Amanda did a lot of walking that day. That's exactly what the doctors and nurses want too, so good all around.

Sometime around 8am, a young man came into the room with a wheelchair. It was time for Amanda's barium swallow. The barium swallow is a procedure that checks your insides for leaks by having you drink some sort of potion in front of an x-ray machine. If you leak, it will show it. Amanda wasn't allowed to swallow anything else until they verified she wasn't leaking. The procedure took about 45 minutes, and I spent that time drinking my breakfast in the parking lot.

It wasn't long after that an attendant showed up with Amanda's brunch. It consisted of a protein drink, sugar free Jell-O, bottled water, and some incredibly nasty beef broth in a cup. Her new assignment was to drink 2 ounces of protein and 3 ounces of water every hour. This assignment was to last the next three weeks.

The rest of the day consisted of nothing but sitting, walking, sipping, peeing (into a bottle), sucking, watching tv, and napping. Amanda was allowed to nap as long as it was in the chair. I was allowed to nap too, and I took advantage of it. Truthfully, she needed very little help from me that day. I was simply moral support. By noon, she was getting up and down out of the chair and walking up and down the halls on her own. As time went on, the pain obviously lessened.

Earlier in the morning, the surgeon had popped in to see how things were progressing. The prognosis was good. Later in the day, the nurse dropped a hint that most bariatric patients go home the day after surgery, and it was up to the surgeon to come in and clear them. She told us the surgeon usually comes in around 5-6 o'clock to do her evaluations. We had a new time to look forward to. Also, around that time, Amanda's sister, newborn nephew Kent, mother, and father were converging on the hospital to visit.

Amanda's family beat the surgeon but not by much. When the doctor came in, her eyes went wide at the vision of the family reunion, but she quickly got down to business. It was a short visit. Amanda was doing great and clear to go home. Everyone was happy, but none more so than Amanda. It had been a long couple of days. It was almost 8pm before she was out of the hospital and back home, but she made it in one piece.

For Amanda, it was over. The surgery was done. All that remained was the recovery. I was happy, proud, and panicked at the same time. Being there for her had given me a unique perspective on my own upcoming procedure. I looked upon it with both excitement and dread.

Chapter 20

The Moment I've Been Waiting For

The week before my surgery was nowhere near as exciting as the week Amanda had before hers. I saw our GP again, just to get his official sign-off. My CT scan came back mostly clear, with only a hint of fatty liver, certainly not enough to prevent me from having the surgery. I had my final visit with the surgeon at the bariatric center, and it was largely forgettable. All in all, it seemed as though the stress leading up to my surgery was over.

Amanda's recovery went well. I think the hardest part for her to endure in the couple of weeks following her surgery was the shots. Each of us were prescribed Lovenox to be taken twice a day for two weeks. Lovenox is a blood thinner that comes in an easy to use stick-yourself-with-a-needle kit for use in the comfort of your own home. Lollipop not included.

I joke, but, in reality, they were easy to give. Each shot was pre-measured and came in a small packet. Once we ripped the package open, administering the shot was as easy as grabbing some flab on the tummy, pinching it up, sticking the needle in, and pushing the plunger. Once the plunger depressed fully, a little safety collar snapped down over the needle. This covered up the sharp bit and forced it out of the body at the same time. From there, it could be thrown away.

Amanda couldn't do it. She used to be an EMT, so it wasn't that she didn't know how or couldn't handle the procedure. She just couldn't deal with sticking a needle into herself. That automatically nominated me to do the sticking for her. No problem, I could stab my wife twice a day. It bruised her terribly, and the angry red and purple blotches lasted for weeks. The medicine also tended to burn at first, but the feeling went away after a few minutes. She and I were glad when the regimen was over.

In addition to the Lovenox, we would both be given Omeprazole to reduce acid reflux and Actigall to prevent gallstones. Both of these medications were to be taken for two months. The Omeprazole wasn't too bad, but the Actigall pills felt like they were the size of a small dog. If you add the extra vitamins, plus our regular medications, it was almost like a meal unto itself.

Thankfully, after just a few days, most of Amanda's surgical gas pain went away, and she felt mostly normal. She was cleared to return to work on the following Monday. We had decided beforehand that she would not take off any days for my surgery. Her job is not as forgiving as mine when it comes to taking leave. While I could afford to take leave for hers, she could not afford to take it for mine. I didn't mind. Maybe it's a man thing, but I wasn't sure I wanted her to see me in a hospital bed too much anyway.

I remember my last full-size meal that week… my last full-size meal ever. My surgery was on Thursday, and I couldn't eat on Wednesday, so it was a Tuesday night. The 5th of December 2017. I had steak. It was glorious. I picked it out at the store and grilled it on our back patio. Nothing crazy, just salt, pepper, some garlic, and a little butter. It was much bigger than six ounces, but I figured it was my last big meal ever so, what the hell? I kept to the official diet though, other than size. There were no carbs to speak of. I think I had some celery with ranch dressing on the side. I might've had a fun-sized candy bar that night. Or two. Maybe.

Amanda, of course, had water and a protein drink. That would be her diet for three weeks, at least officially. My diet for the next day was water, water, and more water. I was supposed to drink at least half my body weight in ounces of water, and that wasn't a little bit. Not having food that day wasn't nearly as hard as I thought it would be, though. With the surgery looming and Amanda basically doing the same thing, I found my willpower to be as high as it ever was, and I didn't cheat even a little bit.

I received a call that day from the hospital to set my schedule. I was hoping for an early time, so I could get it done and over with. They gave me 10 in the morning. Happy with that, I agreed and hung up the phone. I felt glad to be earlier than Amanda's late afternoon time. That would be less time I would need to wait without being able to drink anything. About 15 minutes after I hung up, the hospital called back and told me they had a cancellation and asked if I would like 6 am.

Whoo boy, 6 am? That's like, really early, but if 10 is good then 6 is better right? Sure. I took 6 am. I briefly contemplated why in the world anyone would cancel their surgery the day before, especially after all we'd been through to get to that point, but the thought left almost as soon as it started. It didn't matter why they cancelled, but it meant I had to be up and at the hospital by 5:30. It worked out perfectly because it meant Amanda could drive me to the hospital before work. Otherwise, Dad would've taken me. He didn't mind at all, but this way, he could sleep in and come see me once I was in post-op. Heck, at 6 am, Amanda even had time to go back with me into pre-op and, hopefully, see Lee again.

The bariatric center nurse had instructed Amanda and me to make sure we got a bottle of special body soap to prepare for the surgery. The night before, we were to shower as normal but without shampoo, conditioner, or normal body soap of any kind. Instead, we had to use the special soap. The special soap wasn't much like soap. Instead, it was like a slightly thicker version of hand sanitizer. I did my best to get it to lather, but it was a losing battle.

The nurse's instructions were to put clean sheets on the bed, get a good night's sleep, and shower again in the morning with the special soap. Somehow, I managed a few hours of sleep that night, but I lost the battle with lathering the soap again. It didn't matter. I felt clean and ready to go. We arrived at the hospital right around 5:30 am.

My check-in process was identical to the one Amanda went through, apart from billing. They never bothered to talk about money. After all, I was at my out of pocket maximum for the year. It occurred to me that all the fighting I'd done throughout the last few months regarding our timeline had just paid off. Because I was having the surgery done before the end of the year, our insurance was paying for it in full. It felt good.

I received my armband, and we took another trek to the most depressing surgical waiting room in the universe. Even at 5:45 in the morning, there was not an available seat in front of the television. Since I was the first bariatric surgery of the day, it did not take long for me to be called back. By 6:20, I was giving Lee a big handshake and a smile. He welcomed me back, showed me to my pre-op stall, and checked in with Amanda to see how she was doing after her surgery.

My pre-op procedure was almost identical to the one Amanda had gone through a week earlier, right down to the double pair of socks. The biggest difference for me was that I had to have my abdomen shaved. That was weird. I'm a pretty hairy guy, except for my forehead, which is receding like a shelf full of condoms during an extended power outage. Having a male nurse use a female electric razor on my manly, if a bit jiggly, tummy was a bit strange. The feeling afterwards was even stranger. It was... drafty.

It wasn't long after my bearded belly was bared that an astonishing cavalcade of nurses and doctors began. This was the part I missed for Amanda's surgery while I was off getting my CT scan. The actual surgeon came in, wearing street clothes, and made sure I was doing ok. Then, I met the surgical nurse, the same one that walked Amanda back. She told me I'd be seeing her again soon. Next was another surgical nurse, who told me they would take good care of me. Last was a very disinterested anesthesiologist, who described how he would knock me out like he was reading instructions for programming a VCR.

Each of the doctors or nurses acknowledged Amanda, except for the anesthesiologist. They were all excited to see her again and wanted to know how she was doing. Each left happy and satisfied that she was doing well.

When the time finally came, the first surgical nurse met me in my stall and helped me up out of the bed. They put the little paper shower cap on me and told me it was time to walk into surgery. She asked if I had any other questions and made sure I was ready. I was. I wanted to get the whole thing done and over with. I was excited for it but mostly just tired of everything. Don't get me wrong, it was a happy day and wasn't something I regretted getting into, but it had been one of the most tiring experiences of my life. Part of my happiness was the knowledge that, once it was done, it could not be denied or taken away from me. I was ready.

Amanda and I acted out the same ritual as before her surgery, only in reverse. We kissed, told each other we loved each other, and waved our goodbyes. I found out later that she took all my stuff, including my Sucky McSuckface, and retreated to the waiting room. There, she met Dad and gave him the scoop before she went off to work. Dad would now be my waiting room representative. Later in the morning, Mom would arrive and be his waiting room buddy.

The nurse and I walked arm in arm into the surgical area. I'd never been in this part of the hospital, and it felt exceedingly sterile and a bit lonely. In the pre-op room, there were people everywhere, coming and going, always busy. Once we walked through the big double doors into the surgical hallway, the feeling was eerie, almost too quiet. The nurse and I made small talk during the walk, and I mentioned a memory I had of walking down my high school hallway with a group of friends, arm in arm, doing the 'wizard walk' from the Wizard of Oz. You know the one, where they're skipping and singing down the yellow brick road.

It was a mistake to mention it. She immediately asked me to show her. She had a sly little grin on her face. She knew what I was talking about but wanted me to skip down the hallway to my surgery. I was wearing a funny paper shower cap, two pairs of grippy socks, a hospital gown, massaging leg bladders, and absolutely nothing else. I was also hooked to an IV line and my arm was hooked into the arm of an older, but very pretty, nurse. I was also fat, much fatter than I had been in high school the last time I attempted to wizard walk. That's the point of the surgery, remember?

It didn't matter. There was nothing for it but to give it a go and get through it. I kicked out my right foot and started to skip, just a little bit. She laughed and joined. We awkwardly skipped five or six steps down the hallway and then, mercifully, we were done. I'm sure Judy Garland would've been shocked and appalled at the mockery we made of it, but it didn't matter. I was smiling despite myself. I knew the nurse had seen an opportunity to lighten the mood and took it, and even though I felt a little manipulated, I didn't care. It gave me something to look back on and laugh about.

I barely had time to register these thoughts before we arrived at the operating theatre. It was huge! The room was far larger than I expected. Everything I knew about operating rooms I knew from television. They were never this big on TV. It was also incredibly bright and incredibly busy. The nurse and anesthesiologist I met earlier were already there, prepping and setting things up. I didn't have a chance to take it all in before my nurse escort ushered me to the operating table. It was nothing like I imagined, either.

Above the table, mounted to the ceiling, sat a huge light. This I recognized from TV. It was hooked to an arm that articulated on several joints and looked like it might be as bright as the sun. The table reminded me far more of a torture device than an operating table. It wasn't very wide and was clearly made of metal. There was a foot rest looking thing of some sort on the foot end and an uncomfortable looking headrest on head end. On either side, just below the headrest, were long metal arms that swung out on hinges. As it sat when I first saw it, it would've made a cross if I were looking from above.

In front of it sat a tiny little stool. Clearly, the stool was an afterthought. I was amused to think our surgeon had to find a little stool for her patients to use to climb onto a table that most folks would be lifted onto from a bed. I wasn't sure how

I was going to navigate everything with my gown and IV lines, but somehow, I managed to climb up and onto the table. I adjusted myself to fit into the headrest. The footrest was too far away to use. What happened next was like being the car in an Indianapolis 500 pit stop.

The nurses and anesthesiologist descended on me. One nurse took the footrest and pushed it up against the soles of my feet. Oh, so it wasn't a footrest; it was a sort of clamp to keep me from sliding down the table. The other nurse grabbed my left arm and placed it on the hinged part of the table. Strapping my arm down, she asked me to adjust a little and swung the whole contraption down toward my side once I was in the right position. The other nurse began doing the same to my other arm and had me do a few adjustments to my position. I didn't know what the anesthesiologist was doing exactly, except that he had hooked my IV tube up to something and was behind me to the lef...

Blackness.

No breathing into a respirator. No counting back from ten. No grogginess or sleepiness. Just there one moment and not the next. I had a dream. It was short. I don't remember it.

Chapter 21

Pain, Drugs, and Walk n' Roll

I awoke groggily in the post-op recovery room, feeling like a pack of wild dogs had played hopscotch on my tummy. That is to say, it hurt, but not as much as I was expecting. I couldn't tell if my overall discomfort was because of the anesthetic wearing off, all the equipment I was tied into, or the fallout pain of the surgery. In what little bit of my brain was firing, I figured it was a combination of all those things.

The nurse, realizing I had finally joined the land of the living once again, fetched a cup of ice. As she handed it to me, she told me that my father, currently in the waiting room, would be with me soon. The more consciousness I gained, the more I realized just how dry my mouth was and how much my stomach hurt. I could feel the gas inside trying to find a place to park. The gas pain was brutal and persistent, but I felt as though it could not possibly be as bad as what Amanda experienced. Her pain tolerance tends to be far higher than mine, and my pain didn't even seem close to the amount of pain she let on, let alone actually experienced.

Instead, my largest concern was my mouth. It was dry but more than that. The word dry does not adequately convey the complete and total lack of moisture that was occurring. I would've gladly stuck my head into a bucket of sand to quench the barren, anhydrous wasteland that was my oral cavity. It felt like whatever drugs they were giving me could've desiccated an elephant and its entire lineage back to the stone-age.

Ice was like mana from heaven. I greedily stuck a plastic spoon into the Styrofoam cup full of the stuff and slowly maneuvered it into my mouth. The sweet cool flow of moisture immediately running over my tongue and down my throat made me feel somewhat normal again. I forgot about my mouth for a moment and was able to focus more on how I felt in general. Sore.

Everything was sore. My stomach area was extra sore, but that was to be expected. I looked around the room and mused that, somehow, they had managed to stick me in the exact same post-op bay where they put Amanda a week earlier. As the minutes ticked on, my brain became less fuzzy. It would take me probably an hour or more to be completely all there, but after just five or ten minutes, I was awake enough to hold my own cup of ice.

Dryness. Again. Immediately after the ice in my mouth melted, things went dry again. I couldn't believe how drastic it was, though this time, there was a slightly sticky residue left behind. Somehow, that made it worse. I scrambled as much as I could, considering my condition, to get another piece in my mouth. Just as before, it was a little piece of frozen heaven. This struggle between periods of sucking ice and dry mouth persisted until I could drink actual water the next morning. Even then, the dry mouth feeling would last for days.

Dad finally found his way back to me and took a seat in the chair next to the bed. He told me what the surgeon told him; the surgery was a complete success. She repaired my hernia, and there were no issues. Dad told me how proud of me he was and that he loved me. I could also see the recognition in his eyes… he'd been laying right where I was a few years before.

He had brought my Sucky McSuckface, and I reluctantly gave it a try. I was shocked how weak I was. I could barely move the little plunger up by 10 or 20 points, but the nurse told me I was doing well and to keep it up. For the next 20 or 30 minutes, that was the routine. Ice, suck, nap, Ice, suck, nap.

As time went on, my pain began to grow. The painkillers were wearing off.

Painkillers and anesthetics did some strange things to my memory. My recollections of the time immediately after my surgery are fuzzy and a bit off, so I don't remember exactly when everything took place and in what order. Just like with my EGD, I only remember exact details when I'm reminded of them by someone else. I leaned heavily on my wife and parents to help me recall what happened in the hours following my procedure.

While Dad was still with me, Amanda called to see how I was doing. I let her know everything was fine and tried to sound like I was in less pain than I actually was. Like her, I didn't have a drain put in my abdomen for the air, so that was one less thing to worry about. She told me she loved me, was proud of me, and would see me during her lunch in about an hour. I looked forward to it.

Not long after the phone call, Dad went back to the waiting room, so Mom could come back and see me. She sat down and asked all the questions a loving mother should. How was I doing? How did I feel? Was I happy it was over? I was good, I had some pain, and yes, I was glad it was done. My answers were brief, mostly because of my general soreness and overall fatigue.

Even so, I wanted to walk. I remember the nurse telling Amanda the best way to resolve pain was to walk. My nurse, a different one, told me the same thing. I wanted to get up and walk as soon as possible and with as little help as I could manage. I didn't need any help. I got this. I managed to swing my legs over the side of the bed, just as the nurse became incredibly busy with a new patient. I waited. I had no choice. I was hooked to every machine imaginable.

Soon, it became clear the nurse was not going to return in time to take advantage of my gumption, so Mom helped me back down into the bed. I grumbled a bit about my hookups and waited for the nurse. It wasn't long after my attempted walk that Amanda arrived for her lunch break. She swapped with Mom as my post-op buddy. Just about as soon as she did, the nurse was finally ready to get me up and walking.

I rolled over to the edge of the bed once again, but this time, the nurse was there to unhook me. Once I had swung out of the bed, Amanda walked me around the room, just as I had done for her. I managed to go farther than she did, just to say to myself that I could, and shuffled back to the bed. I did it mostly on my own, even though Amanda was there holding my arm, just in case. I felt very happy with that... I guess it's the little things.

Mirroring Amanda's procedure, after my walk, it was time to wait for my room. Amanda visited for as long as she could, even returning a little late to work. I don't think anyone cared, considering the circumstances. Once she left me, I was the lone ranger for a little while until the room was ready. That was fine by me. I love my family a great deal but having a short period of personal time to reflect and regroup was nice.

It wasn't until about 2pm that they started preparing to wheel me up to my room. I couldn't wait. My own room meant freedom and privacy just as it had for Amanda, at least as much as can be had as a patient in a hospital. When I arrived in my room, I found my parents waiting with one of the nurses assigned to that floor.

Turns out that Mom and Dad had been waiting a while and already had some issues with the room. It was bare. There was no equipment or amenities normally associated with a hospital room, other than a small recliner and the ubiquitous tiny television. It wasn't until after I'd been wheeled in that they started moving IV stands, oxygen monitors, air compressors, and other miscellaneous medical doodads into the room. Mom was not impressed.

Her mood did not improve when the nurse immediately started asking me the standard series of medical questions once I was wheeled in. The tires on my hospital bed hadn't even had a chance to cool down before she started in with all the same questions I'd heard a dozen times before.

What's your full name? What's your birthday? Are you allergic to any medications? What state where you born in? Have you or a loved one ever been convicted of a felony involving a stuffed buffalo, easy cheese, and a container of that orange goop mechanics use to clean their hands... you know, the gritty stuff?

When we all started looking at her like she'd grown a second head, she explained the hospital computers don't talk to each other. That's why she had to ask all the questions again. I couldn't believe it. Here I was, barely out of surgery, and I was playing twenty questions with Nurse Ratchet because some IT guy somewhere was still using an abacus.

She asked me my pain level, and, like a dumbass, I was honest.

"About a six."

She raised an eyebrow, "A six? That's very good. Usually patients right out of surgery are much higher."

The way the nurses always word this question is as follows: "On a scale of one to ten, one being no pain and ten being the worst pain you've ever experienced, how bad is your pain level right now?"

In my ignorance, I thought back to the worst pain I'd ever experienced. It was my gout attack years earlier when I was reduced to wheeling around the house in a computer chair. During that attack, even something as simple as a bed sheet resting on my foot would send me shrieking into a pillow. I have read online where folks say a gout attack is second only to child birth in pain intensity. My post-op pain was nothing compared to that.

It was still quite painful, though. Painful enough that I wanted painkillers. Badly. I reconsidered, "Well, actually it's an eight right this moment. It was a six earlier, but I think my last batch of painkillers is wearing off."

Mom smiled. She knew I'd learned my lesson. The nurse raised her eyebrow again. "Ok, well, it looks like we can give you another dose in about a half-hour or so."

If you want painkillers, always overstate your pain level. If you're a five, make it a seven. If you're at seven, make it nine. If you're below six or so, they'll pretty much just tell you to suck it up and stop being a sissy. And walk. Always walk. I'm sure they would've told me to drink a lot of water too, were I able to drink.

Painkillers are a guarded and sensitive subject in the hospital. At least they were in the hospital Amanda and I were in. Nurses were reluctant to talk about them and very rarely volunteered to administer them. I suppose it's a symptom of the ongoing opioid problem in the US, but it's a real pain in the ass for folks in the hospital that actually need them. Asking a nurse for painkillers almost always resulted in the same conversation.

"Nurse, can I get some painkillers? It really hurts."

"Well, we already gave you some a few hours ago. On a scale of one to ten, one being no pain and ten being the worst pain you've ever experienced, how bad is your pain level right now?"

"Twenty-two"

"That doesn't seem that bad. We had a patient the other day that was over a hundred, and they didn't get any. I will see what I can do. In the meantime, get up and walk."

Ok, so that might be an exaggeration, but the nurse always told me they'd "just given me some," and asked, "On a scale of one to ten, one being no pain and ten being the worst pain you've ever experienced, how bad is your pain level right now?" They would always finish with, "I'll have to get approval from the head nurse. I'll see what I can do. In the meantime, the best way to get rid of the pain is to walk."

Mom and I did walk, not long after the nurse finished her line of questioning and reluctantly agreed to administer more drugs. Dad gave his knees a rest back in the room. That first walk out of my own room was painful, but nowhere near as bad as Amanda's had been. I remember Amanda's first walk out of her room and down the corridor. I remember the crying and the look of agony on her face. My walk with Mom was slow and painful, but I had nowhere near the gas pain Amanda did. Still, it was bad enough to comment. I did so once we reached the window at the end of the hall.

"You know Mom, I think I understand something now," I said, looking out the window.

"Oh?" She paused, waiting for me to finish my thought.

"Not that I want to die or anything, but I think I can understand why people sometimes want to kill themselves when they're in constant pain with no end in sight," I explained. "I know this pain will end in the next few days, a week at most, and I can deal with it, but if I knew I'd have to live with it the rest of my life... I don't know if I could."

She smiled a very motherly smile and nodded. Mom had always taught me to reserve judgement on folks who killed themselves. She always said, "You have no idea what they've gone through. Nobody has. Every person is different, and every pain is different. Don't ever think you wouldn't do it if you were in their shoes... you just don't know."

We took the rest of our trip, and I made my way back with very little fanfare. I was given a slight nod of approval when I meandered by the nurse's station. I found out, as my walks over the next day or so continued, that a cursory nod from the nurses was almost customary during a post-surgical walk.

Back in the room, I spent most of my time in the little recliner. A nurse had started to change the bedsheets but somehow decided not to finish. Perhaps there were no clean sheets. In any case, the bed sat there, barren. The mattress was ugly, vinyl, and the color of an overripe eggplant. Not anything I wanted to lay on.

After work, sometime around 5:30 or so, Amanda came by to see how I was doing. The four of us visited for a bit, and eventually, Amanda and Mom took me on another foray into the exciting world of hospital corridors. Each walk got a little easier, and by this time, Mom and Amanda were mostly just moral support. I was pretty much doing all the walking on my own.

My parents said their loves and goodbyes sometime around 8 that night. Amanda stuck around a bit longer, and it was really the first time since the surgery we had time alone. She took the opportunity to ask me something personal.

"Have you peed yet?"

"What?" I asked, a little surprised. She wasn't usually this candid about bathroom habits.

"Have you peed? I only ask because I never felt like I had to go after the surgery. My body never gave me the signal like I had to pee. At one point I just tried, and, sure enough, I had to go."

"Really?" I was amused. I certainly hadn't felt the need to go since I woke up from the operation. I suppose it couldn't hurt to see if my plumbing still worked.

We were each made to pee in a bottle after our surgeries. I think it was so they could measure our liquid intake and output. Either that or someone in that hospital had a fetish. In any case, it made me especially glad to be a man. Peeing in a bottle was practically an instinct. To my shock and amusement, I did have to go and not just a little bit. Normally, a flow like the one I unleashed that night would've had me hopping up and down and doing a little dance. For some reason, it was like my body didn't even care. Thankfully, the pee pee dance feeling did return after a few days.

Before Amanda went home for the night, she helped me out of my drafty hospital gown and into some normal person pajamas. It made me feel much more civilized and human, so I was grateful. We said our goodbyes. Amanda let me know she would be by during lunch and after work the next day. Hopefully after work, she said, they'd let me go home, and it would all be over. I hoped that too, but I wasn't worried. I felt like I was doing great, all things considered.

Once Amanda was gone and I was the lone ranger again, one of the nurses dutifully informed me I should be walking as much as possible, at least four times an hour while awake. She asked me to let them know if I wanted to walk, so they could get me unplugged.

If walking meant less pain, then I was all for it. Besides being the only way to get the gas bubbles to move around and dissipate, it was pretty much the only thing to do. There was a television, but it was boring. It was also uncomfortable to hang out in the chair, so it wasn't long before I wanted to walk on my own for the first time. I hit the call button on the funky remote / bed control / call button thingy to call a nurse.

The nurse that came was much younger than the one who told me to call for assistance. I told her I wanted to walk.

"Ok, great. You can go ahead whenever you're ready. You don't need a nurse to unplug you."

Oh, ok. Um. Right.

After she left, I assessed my situation. I had a good idea of how to unhook myself due to the walks I'd taken earlier.

Oxygen monitor. That was a little doohickey that clamped on to my finger. Unclamp it, no problem.

What about the IV? Well, it had to come with me. It was on a stand that had wheels, so it became my new best friend for the next day and a half. It plugged into the wall with some kind of adapter that unhooked near the machine. I gave it a tug. The adapter unhooked, and the machine kept running. A little battery icon and number appeared. Good deal. IV taken care of.

Now for my leg massagers. I needed them unplugged from their compressor, so I could walk. Air hoses connected them to the machine, so I found the little twist off connectors. Just twist 'em off, no problem.

Except I couldn't reach. They were way the hell down by my feet and bending over made my insides feel squishy in a bad kind of way. I found that I could reach the one on my right without much effort, so I unhooked it. The massager on my left leg was a different story. Somehow, either because they were made different or installed differently, the hose connection sat further down.

I was a man. (Grunt grunt) I did what I had to do. I wasn't going to go yelling for a nurse, especially after a nurse had clearly told me I could do it myself. I bent down, held my breath, endured the squishiness, grimaced heroically, and completely failed to unhook the hose. It took two more attempts, but I finally managed to unhook the bastard. I sat up again, breathing sweet air and panting. I needed more ice to wet my mouth, but I was free. I grabbed Mr. IV Cart and we were on our way to my first solo adventure in hospital corridor land.

Back in the room, all I could do was sit in the chair, watch television, check my phone, and suck on ice. It was imperative that I kept my ice cup from running out or melting completely, or my mouth would, once again, become cracked and arid like some kind of Saharan wasteland. I would give Sucky a workout whenever I remembered, which was not always as often as I should. Every hour or so, a nurse would come in and make sure I wasn't dead by checking the machines and giving me a brief visual inspection. I couldn't wait until it was time for bed. I was exhausted. At some point, a nurse finally came in to replace my sheets.

The hospital bed was uncomfortable, and I don't like to sleep on my back, but I didn't have a choice on either count. At least I wasn't wearing the gown. I fell asleep sometime around 10pm and woke up once or twice during the night when nurses came in to check off their clipboard and verify that I was, in fact, still alive. As the night wore on, the painkillers wore off. Soreness began to creep back into my chest and abdomen and join the gas pain, which never really left. Gas pain, by the way, is not solved by painkillers. It doesn't go away; you just get used to it.

When I woke up at 4 am, I knew I was done sleeping. The discomfort of the bed, coupled with my increasing soreness, made the thought of continuing to sleep almost unbearable. I got up and moved to the chair, where I snapped on the television and dozed in and out for the rest of the morning. A nurse came in around 6 to do the rounds and let me know I was no longer allowed in the bed. Fine by me. I asked about painkillers to deal with my painful abdomen. I received the same talk as before, but, thankfully, the nurse capitulated.

Light was coming in through the window. Morning had arrived. I couldn't wait until the transport kid came to my room with the wheelchair to take me to my barium swallow, so I could be cleared for fluids. I asked the nurse when I could expect to see him.

"They usually come up around 10 o'clock." It was 6:30. I still had hours to go.

Luckily for me, she was wrong. The transport kid glided into my room right around 8. I was ecstatic. Finally, the next phase was happening. Not only did it give me something to do, but it meant I could start drinking fluid again, provided I passed the swallow. He helped me into the wheelchair, threw a blanket around me because, "It gets cold down there," and wheeled me downstairs to the imaging area. We ended our trip in a small x-ray room that somehow looked like it belonged in the basement of a high school.

The transport kid told me to sit and wait for the lab technician and the doctor. His name was Dr. Smiley. No shit. I don't know what Dr. Smiley was doing, but he was certainly busy with something, because I waited quite a while. I was glad for the blanket but wished heartily for ice. My mouth had turned to desert again, and there was nothing I could do but smack my lips and roll my inadequately lubricated tongue around my mouth in dry sticky impotency. I sat.

After what felt like an eternity, the technician came in and started fiddling with the x-ray machine. He tipped it from laying down to standing up and instructed me to stand between the bed of the machine and the imaging plate. I was happy to have something to do other than sit, so I obliged heartily. He handed me a cup of liquid, my barium swallow. My mouth would've watered, but it was incapable. I wanted so badly to drink, but I had to wait for Dr. Smiley.

It wasn't long before the Dr. arrived and finished getting the machine ready. There was a monitor directly behind my head to the right, and I found I could see it pretty well if I stretched my neck around that way. Neither the Dr. nor the technician seemed to be bothered by my movement, so I looked on, fascinated. I was seeing a real-time view of the inside of my body. Apparently, I would be able to see the liquid moving through. Cool!

The Dr. instructed me to take a sip. Finally! This was the moment I'd been waiting for. My mouth was so dry... a drink of anything would be better than nothing. I eagerly brought the cup to my lips and took a sip.

I was wrong. This. This could be worse than nothing. It was horrid, like old differential fluid mixed with used sandpaper grit. It coated the inside of my mouth, eagerly filling the torrid void, and slid down the back of my throat. In one of life's great ironies, the fluid, somehow, did almost nothing to quench the dryness. Instead, it simply coated everything with an awful gooey texture. I was so focused on dealing with the taste and texture that I almost forgot to look at the screen.

Almost forgot. I should've forgot. I did look, though, and saw something horrifying. A dark blotch moved from the top of the screen down into what looked like my chest cavity. It moved in fits and spurts, and then, suddenly, shot almost horizontally to the right of the screen and then continued its journey down. My mind reeled.

"Oh no!" I thought, "A leak!" It must be, shooting out like that.

"Again," Dr. Smiley instructed, "take another sip."

He didn't sound concerned. That was a good sign. I braced myself and did what I had to do. The cup was now half empty. I prayed that I didn't need to finish it.

Looking back at the screen, again, I saw the same fit, spurt, and shoot pattern that I saw before. I quickly glanced at the Dr. then the technician. Neither seemed to have a care in the world.

"Looks normal to me," the Dr. concluded. "We'll take a closer look in the back, but I don't see any issues." To say I was relieved is an understatement. The technician let the transport kid know I was ready to go back to my room.

I've never been so happy to see an ice cube in my entire life.

It wasn't long before an attendant entered the room with a tray full of liquids. My breakfast was a little late by normal standards, probably around 10am by that time, but I didn't care. It meant my barium swallow turned out fine, and there were no leaks to be found. It also meant I could finally use something other than ice to moisten my mouth. On the tray sat a bottle of water, a cup of chicken broth, a container of room temperature Jell-O, and a huge bottle of protein drink. The protein drink was orange flavored and colored to match.

From that moment on, for the next month, I was required to drink, and record, at least 2oz of protein and 3oz of water every hour. For my convenience, they also gave me a small stack of one-ounce plastic cups. I set about getting my water intake right away. I filled up one of the cups with the bottled water and judged to myself that I could take about half of it at a time. That was far less than I would normally drink and should be safe. It's just water.

The water was like paradise to my dry mouth and throat. I couldn't believe how wonderful a simple drink of water could be, but unfortunately, my euphoria didn't last long. Since I hadn't had a drink in over 36 hours, my stomach was completely empty, and I could feel the water sliding down my esophagus. Once it hit the point where my esophagus met my new stomach, a shot of pain gripped my insides like a vice. The pain was raw and completely unexpected. My eyes snapped shut and a grimace escaped my lips. What the hell was that?

I tried again with the second half of my ounce. The pain was almost the same, though not quite as intense. It felt like there was a huge open cold sore down there that had a tiny throat gnome rolling around in it. The pain lasted for as long as it took for the liquid to pass through. I assumed it was simply a result of the surgery, and it would go away over time. As I continued to drink my liquids and mark my progress, the pain continued as well. It was something I got used to. At least it only happened when I drank.

The orange protein drink wasn't great but different than water or ice, so acceptable. It certainly wasn't as bad as the barium swallow had been. The pain was the same, no matter what I drank. I tried the broth. Cold. Nasty. Not worth the agony.

My day boiled down to napping in the chair, watching television, walking every fifteen to thirty minutes, giving Sucky some attention now and then, and dealing with trying to swallow liquid. Occasionally, I would take a bathroom break which, oddly, was almost like a vacation from everything else.

Amanda stopped in during her lunch hour to check on me and take me on a walk. By that time, I was walking on my own routinely. I needed no help at all, and it was almost like a stroll through the park, other than dragging Mr. IV with me the whole time. We talked about my swallowing and how interesting it was that she had worse gas pain than I did, but I had worse swallowing pain than she did. After our walk, Amanda went back to work.

Dad stopped by around 1 o'clock to see how I was doing. I asked him about the swallowing pain. It was getting worse, somehow. Looking back, I think it was painkillers wearing off.

He indicated he didn't have any after his surgery and wondered aloud if maybe it was my hernia repair. Of course! That made total sense. The hernia was at the top of my stomach near my esophagus, and if she had removed it, there would be a wound there that was raw and sore. I felt much better, at least mentally. The pain of swallowing had never been so bad.

I distinctly remember the worst of it. I figure my painkillers had almost totally worn off by that point, but I could do nothing but continue my required regimen. In the space of about two hours in the early afternoon the day after surgery, I experienced the third worst pain of my life, right after the pain from my gout flare-up years earlier and watching The Astronaut Farmer. Taking even a moderate swallow caused me to double over with agony, and I found myself scrunching my face and actually shaking my clenched fist in an effort to relieve it. Each time, the pain lasted for only a few seconds, which made the effort just tolerable enough to continue.

When a nurse came in to check on me, I told her about the pain, and we went through the painkiller talk. Once the painkillers were administered, the pain subsided a great deal. It was still uncomfortable to swallow, but far less so than before. Thankfully, my swallowing pain would only continue for a few days afterwards and then disappear. It never manifested itself again, at least not as badly as while my father was visiting that afternoon.

Later that night, I went on to ask the surgeon about the pain and mention Dad's thought about the hernia. She agreed completely. The pain was normal and should subside after just a few days. In the meantime, they were prescribing some liquid courage in the form of hydrocodone. Otherwise, she told me, I looked great and was doing great. She saw no reason to keep me at the hospital. Amanda was just getting off work around the time I got my clearance to leave. The whole operation went like clockwork, and I was packing up when Amanda arrived to take me home.

Just like her before me, I was done. The surgery was successful, and I now had an itty-bitty stomach. I wasn't looking forward to the next few weeks of liquid diet, but I was overjoyed that both of us were through to the other side. Not only that, but we managed to sneak it in before the end of the year, saving us countless thousands of dollars. All that was left now was to recover. I didn't know it then, but my pain wasn't quite over. The third worst was, yes, but the fourth worst pain of my life was yet to come.

Chapter 22

Things Your Doctor Won't Tell You

When having a procedure like bariatric surgery, there's a lot of information thrown at you all at once. We received instructions on how and what to eat, how and what to drink, and what kind of lifestyle changes we would need to undergo to maximize our weight loss and health after the surgery. It's inevitable that some things slip through the cracks, and other things aren't talked about simply because they're either too personal or too specific to individual situations.

One thing that slipped through the cracks for me, or maybe it was left out entirely, was the size of the sips I needed to take immediately after the surgery. I felt like a half ounce sip was small enough at the time, but, in reality, even a half ounce was probably too big. Before the surgery, I was the kind of guy that would fill up a twenty-ounce glass of water and chug the whole thing down without taking a breath, so something the size of a half-ounce seemed incredibly tiny to me. Taking sips too large probably contributed to the pain I felt while drinking in the hospital and the few days afterwards.

Another thing that nobody told us was just how to drink those small amounts. I did some research, after everything was over, and found that a human being's natural instinct is to breathe in through the nose while drinking. This allows the body to continue to breathe while the mouth is busy, making sure we don't all drown or choke to death. Of course, I continued to do this as I drank my little one-ounce cups, slowly ingesting a little bit of air with each sip.

There's another thing that happened to me, specifically, immediately following the surgery. It's something I suspect they didn't talk about because it's extremely personal and specific to each person.

I couldn't fart.

In fact, it was like that entire part of my body just said, "the hell with it," and shut down completely. My intestines didn't know what my stomach had done to deserve being cut like that, but they weren't about to make the same mistake. They decided inaction was the best course to take. Besides, it wasn't like they were doing me any good anyway, right? I hadn't eaten anything in days and what little liquid I took in could be handled by my bladder. My bladder didn't seem deterred by my stomach's trauma in the least, so at least that was something.

My bladder, however, wanted nothing to do with all the air I was ingesting. My stomach refused to give it up, citing pain and suffering. So, the job of ridding my body of air was down to my intestines, who seemed to be on some kind of strike. This was definitely the case of death by a thousand gulps, and I didn't even notice until my second night home. Right around bedtime, I started having intestinal cramps. By midnight, the cramping was so bad I had to get up and walk around. By one, I was mixing fiber powder with water. By two, I was drinking milk of magnesia. By three, I was desperate and pounding Mira Lax as fast as I could get it in.

The bariatric center called this progression of medication the 'constipation pathway.' No shit. That was a poop joke, by the way. Stay classy!

By three thirty, the pain was so bad I couldn't stand it anymore. I didn't want to take the painkillers they'd given me, but I didn't have a choice. After a dose of hydrocodone, the cramping finally subsided to a level where I could doze for a while. I sat on the couch in our living room just in case my intestines decided to wake up before I did. I needn't have worried. When I woke up a few hours later, they were grumbling like an oncoming freight train but still had no desire to deflate.

Eventually, by late morning, things down there were moving again. I'll not get into the specifics... I've already had one poop joke too many, but for the sake of those of you who might be having the surgery, I will say one thing. No, that's not roofing tar, and yes, it's normal.

After about three days, I began to feel like my old self again. It took about that long for the soreness to wear off and the feeling of swallowing horny toads to go away completely. The bariatric center charged us with keeping a meticulous journal of our liquid intake, but by the third day, I was just drinking when I felt like it and marking the boxes at the end of the day. Amanda started doing the same after her third day. Both of us were careful to drink the right amounts over the whole day but drinking by ounce by hour felt a little ridiculous.

After a week, I had my follow-up class with the nurse and visit with the doctor. The class was simply a reminder of how to eat during stage two, which would be after three weeks of recovery. My visit with the surgeon went well. My incisions were healing nicely, and there was no sign of infection. Amanda's visit had been largely the same.

We fell into a pretty regular routine after that. Amanda was ahead of me by about a week when it came to our diet restrictions, but... to be completely honest... we didn't follow them very closely. We had done a lot of reading online, and each of us had friends who had gone through the procedure. The online diets and our friends' diets both backed up one fact; our surgeon was incredibly strict.

Our official diet called for nothing but liquid until day 21. That included Jell-O and pudding, but only if it was sugar free. After day 21 and up to day 60, we were only allowed items from a very short list of 'soft' food, such as baked white fish, Greek yogurt, unsweetened applesauce, very soft cooked vegetables, very soft cheese, and cottage cheese. After day 60, we could graduate to chicken, pork, and other things that were softish. There was to be no red meat until after six months, and no raw vegetables for at least that long. Nuts and crunchy things that were hard to digest were reserved for a year out, as was alcohol and caffeine of any kind.

We were to stay under 25 carbs a day for at least six months and could never have potatoes, rice, corn, beans, bread, or any other carby food. Ever.

Amanda and I both thought that was bullshit. Why the hell had we gone through all this, just so we could be on the same damned diet as before? No. We went through this, so we could eat the foods we like, but in smaller quantities. They told us bariatric surgery is a tool, so use the tool to eat healthier. Eating healthier, in part, is eating less… especially in America. We did want to use it to eat less but not like a bludgeon to make our lives miserable by not eating stuff we like.

I think the reason our surgeon was so strict is because people are stupid. Ok, that's mean. What I should say is that people, especially where we're located, sometimes have a hard time following directions. I think the strictness of the diet and the craziness of all the logging reflect that. For example, without water, you get dehydrated, right? Especially when you're not eating anything. During my one-week class, one of the ladies admitted she wasn't drinking much water. Her excuse was that she had been brought up in a family where drinking in front of others was rude, and she was almost never alone. That's why they made us mark those dumb little sheets to prove we were doing it. It's her fault.

Another girl in the class admitted to not taking her vitamins. When you don't eat food, you don't get much nutrition. Vitamins help deal with that. We were required to take two humongous chewable vitamins a day. They were disgusting, but we did what we had to. Except this girl didn't because they didn't taste good. She decided they weren't that important and stopped taking them. I'm sure the office is working on a vitamin log to make sure we all take our vitamins right now.

We heard another story about a local guy who had the surgery done and just couldn't wait to have some chips and salsa. We're in New Mexico, so that's a big deal around here. He decided it would be ok to have some about four weeks after the surgery. Lo and behold, he didn't chew his tortilla chips enough and cut his sutures. That guy. He's the reason we couldn't have anything more solid than pudding for three weeks.

It's fun to blame folks, but to be fair, I think the surgeon just wanted to give us the best chance of success. Still, Amanda and I did accelerate our timeline as we saw fit. We never did anything I would consider radical or stupid in terms of eating, but both of us were eating cottage cheese by the end of two weeks and chicken well before three months.

It was easy to tell when we'd strayed just a bit too far off the plan for our own good. For each of us, a bit of breaded chicken or a mound of mashed potatoes would sometimes give us pause and make us think twice about cheating. When we found a food that gave our tummies a little trouble, we would re-evaluate and move foods like that back a little in our timeline to try again later.

Doing so seemed to work well. More than once, we moved a food back by about a week, only to try it again and find it gave us very little trouble on the second go around. In this way, we could slowly introduce new things, without stressing ourselves too much. Neither of us ever got sick or felt sick to our stomachs.

There were a couple of occasions when we felt full enough to be uncomfortable, though. It was amazing how quickly it would happen, and, for both of us, it tended to happen during either a big holiday meal or during a meal that we'd been looking forward to trying again after the surgery. For me, it was a quesadilla made from the lavash bread. I loved that dish, still do, and having it again after surgery was amazing. So amazing that I forgot myself.

I took one bite too many and suffered the consequences. The discomfort, bordering on actual pain, only lasted five or ten minutes, but it was enough to remind me just how small my stomach had become. It probably won't be the last time.

Chapter 23

Life in Itty Bitty Bites

We both went on to recover fully from the procedure. Two months on, each of us feels almost normal again. If I were to listen to the nutritionists at the bariatric center, I'm still only allowed white fish, yogurt, and some types of cheese. In reality, I've had all types of soup, chicken in many different ways, and even slow cooked ribs. I tried peanut butter only two weeks after surgery and began drinking milk again after three... both big no no's if you ask our doctors. I still avoid some of the scarier things, like nuts, raw vegetables, hard fruit, potato chips, and firm red meat, though. I'll give my body more time to heal for those.

Food feels different now. My insides process it differently. I'm not sure how much of the feeling will be permanent, but, at least for now, each new food takes time to get used to. It's almost as if my stomach needs to relearn how to digest things, and everything it hasn't seen since the surgery needs to be studied before it can be digested. The harder things are to digest, the more they need to be studied. Once I've had it a few times though, things seem to be back to normal.

My cravings for food have dropped significantly. I'm guessing it's mostly because I'm missing the ghrelin hormone, but I don't really care why... it's pretty great not feeling like I want to eat all the time. If you told me right now that I'd have to skip dinner tonight, I'd be just fine with it. So long as I had my protein shake so I got the nutrition I needed, I could be ok almost not eating at all. Of course, I'd rather eat because food still tastes good, and I like it, but I don't feel the deprivation I would've felt before the surgery. Had you told me three months ago that I had to skip dinner, I would've told you how to go directly to hell.

I find myself needing to relearn everything about food, especially when it comes to how much I can eat. It's shocking just how little I eat now. My eyes are used to filling up a big plate with food and never finding the end of my stomach. There is no question now; my stomach has an end. After roughly a cup of food, I'm done. It's not a, "Well, I'm satisfied and feel pretty full," kind of done, but more of a, "This will not fit," kind of done. As I reach the end of my capacity, my esophagus starts refusing to move the food into my stomach. This is very uncomfortable but not painful. If I wiggle a little bit or maybe get up and walk around, things will settle, and I'm able to get another bite in.

I think back on our first trip to a fast food joint since the surgery. We decided to stop in at Burger King for a late breakfast. They have a deal where we can each get a breakfast sandwich for just a couple of bucks, and the folks there know how to ring it up as low carb, so we don't get the bread. We each end up with a piece of cheese, a piece of sausage, and a hunk of scrambled egg in a little bowl. The size turns out to be almost perfect for our new tummies.

I remember finishing my modest little breakfast and, looking across the restaurant, I noticed a girl of about twelve pounding down a double Whopper. I was awestruck. Here I was, a grown ass man of almost forty, filled to the brim by a single breadless breakfast sandwich that was typically sold in pairs. This little girl was going to town on her Whopper, and I wondered where on Earth she was putting it. Prior to the surgery, I wouldn't have given her a second thought. Heck, I would've joined her with two double Whoppers of my own. That kind of intake is ridiculous even to think about now. Even if you took off the bread, I couldn't fit a single, let alone a double.

This is both great and incredibly frustrating. It's great because it forces me to stop eating. Not only can I not fit any more food in there, but my mind almost refuses to try. It's a strange feeling, one I never had before the surgery. My body knows when it would be a mistake to put another bite of food in my mouth, even though my brain hasn't got the signal that I'm full. It's like there's a bouncer at the gate between my throat and my stomach, and, at some point, it gets the message that my stomach can't fit any more. Once that happens, it's impossible for me to put food in my mouth. No matter how much I want it, I can tell that my stomach won't let it in.

It's frustrating because I usually do want to eat more. Inevitably, I'm eating something delicious, and suddenly, my stomach bouncer slams the door while I'm mid-chew or have a very enticing bite of something on a fork just waiting to be admitted. Amanda can tell when this happens because my face falls a little bit, and I sit there, impotently, with a forkful of food just waiting for my bouncer to say, "Ok, ok. Room for one more." Sometimes it does, and sometimes it doesn't. When it doesn't, I often get a little angry at myself and feel upset about the surgery. I dream of a time when I could eat more. The feeling only lasts a few seconds, though, before I get the signal that I'm full, and my desire to eat slips away all on its own. It's at this point that my hiccups tend to start.

For some reason, I get hiccups all the time after eating. Prior to the surgery hiccups were rare for me and usually quite viscous. After the surgery I get them all the time following a meal, but they're mild. It's almost like my stomach is trying to kick some food back up my throat but isn't really giving it much effort. They usually last five or ten minutes and dissipate. I'm guessing it's like my body's way of shaking a garbage bin to get the trash to settle. I do that all the time, so I can put off changing the bag, so I can relate.

The worst of it comes when I haven't chewed something enough or if I eat something particularly dry. Of course, I'm not allowed anything like that yet, but I eat it anyway because I know better than the doctors do. In any case, if I eat something like that, often it will get stuck on the way down.

Prior to the surgery, I would wash it down with a big gulp of soda or water. That's not an option now. After the surgery, you don't drink while you're eating, so I have to just sit there and hope the food finds the way to my stomach. Again, it's not painful, but it is uncomfortable. Walking helps. So does chewing first.

My dad told me prior to our surgeries that the doctors don't want you drinking while you eat. That sounded absolutely preposterous to me. I loved drinking while I ate, washing things down, getting some refreshment. The reasons they gave were things like, "If you drink while you're eating, you'll stretch your stomach," and "If you fill up on liquid, you won't get the nutrition you need." I thought all that stuff was hogwash, and I would be damned if I wasn't going to enjoy a nice cool beverage while I ate my dinner, no matter what size my stomach was.

I was wrong. It's not about wanting to drink, and it's not about willpower. It's not about following doctor's orders or even doing what's right for your health. I don't drink while I eat because I can't afford to. Eating after bariatric surgery is like living paycheck to paycheck. Imagine the size of your stomach is like your bank account. The bigger the stomach, the more money you have. Now imagine that food and drink are the bills you pay and the crap you buy. With a large stomach account, you can pay all the bills and buy some nice things for yourself while you're at it. That means you can eat all the food and drink all the drink. With a small stomach account, you can't always pay all your bills, so you pick and choose the most important ones to pay first. If you decide to spend your money on worthless frivolities, then you can hardly pay any of the bills, even if they're important. Likewise, with a small stomach, you can't fill it up with water and still expect to eat anything significant.

Bottom line is, if you want to eat food you like, you ditch the drink to make room. Every sip of drink during a meal is one less bite you can take. It matters when you can only fit a cup of food in a sitting, so I don't drink during meals anymore. It sucks, but the size of my stomach doesn't allow me a choice. It's one or the other, so I choose food during food times and choose to drink during times when there is no food. Food is better. I pay those bills first.

No matter the downsides, I will say it works. Two months after surgery, I've lost close to fifty pounds. Amanda is down at least forty-five. It comes off in weird places. Amanda's lost almost all her weight from her hips. She's looking great, but she's a bit frustrated that it's not really coming off her tummy yet. It means she hasn't really dropped any pants sizes, even though her hips are much thinner. For me, it's come off my face, my arms, my thighs, my tummy, and even my butt. I can knock my knees together now. Just today, I sat with my legs crossed like a woman for the first time in my entire life. That may not seem exciting, but it was for me.

I have a habit of tucking the bottom of my shirt up under my chin when I need to look at my stomach in the mirror. I also do it if I need to use the urinal in a men's room, just to be sure I don't get the bottom of my shirt wet. It's a habit so ingrained that I don't even think about it. I just do it. The other day, I was looking in the mirror, checking out my incisions, when my shirt fell down out of my chin. I shrugged, tucked it back up under there, and resumed checking myself out. It wasn't more than a couple of seconds before it fell again. I wondered what the hell was going on... it was like my ability to do something I'd done all my life suddenly went away. I couldn't understand it at first, but then I realized my chin is smaller. I have to tuck my head down more to hold the shirt up. I've been used to having a big flabby chin, and my brain hasn't yet compensated for the size change. I have to concentrate on using my chin to hold my shirt up now. It's strange, and that's just one example of how things are changing.

I can't speak for Amanda here, but I will say I have more energy. I enjoy playing with our dogs more, and I even take the opportunity to run around the yard a little bit. Exercise is more fun than it used to be. I mean, it still sucks, but it sucks way less. Fifty pounds is a lot of weight I'm not lugging around anymore, and I can feel it when I walk, jog, or even just get up from the couch. I walk a little faster, a little taller, and I feel more pride in myself and my appearance overall. It makes all the no Whopper eating stomach bouncering hiccups worth it. Every new day is now the lightest I've been since I was in grade school, and my future seems brighter. Knowing that Amanda is losing weight too and being able to see it every day, lets me know the future is brighter for both of us and, God willing, our future kids.

I still eat chocolate and sweets on occasion. Amanda and I both have the odd Reese's or small ice cream cup. We even bought a few boxes of Girl Scout Cookies the other day, and we have one or two every now and then. Before the surgery, we would've had four or five each, so that's something. We refuse to deny ourselves the simple things that make us feel normal and make life worth living for us. We don't have sweets every night, but we don't feel guilty when we do have them. We continue to lose weight, even though we cheat.

And that's it, right? That's the whole point. It's true that we're not losing as much as we could be, now that we're both eating regular foods, including foods the nutritionist hates, like mashed potatoes, milk, chocolate, or even crackers. That's a choice we've made, and if we feel like we're not losing fast enough, we'll modify our diet to suit. The ability to eat far less and still feel satisfied is a very powerful tool, and one we're both still learning how to use. For now, I'm extremely happy with our results. As long as the weight keeps dropping, even if it's slow, I'll keep eating things that make me happy, even if the portions are tiny. What I've found is that you don't need a huge portion of something to be satisfied. Take small bites and enjoy the taste. Even with a small stomach, meals can be great, and, even in small amounts, taste can be big.

Chapter 24

Lessons Learned the Hard Way

If you count the time from my first visit with the nutritionist in the bariatric center to my one-month post-op appointment, it took just under twenty months to get my sleeve gastrectomy done. In that time, I went from not caring about what I ate to thinking about every single bite. Having the procedure done with my wife was one of the most interesting and memorable experiences of my life, and I'm incredibly happy we could improve our health and share the ride together. I couldn't imagine doing it alone.

If I had it all to do over again, I wouldn't hesitate. There were many ups and many downs, of course. Many more downs than I expected, to be honest, but it was all worth it and then some. If you or a loved one are contemplating bariatric surgery, I want you to know I give the gastric sleeve my full endorsement. It's been a blessing to Amanda and me, and I'm sure it will continue to bless us with weight loss and health far into the future. It has done so for my father, as it has done for many good friends.

The title of this book is probably a little misleading, but I wanted it to grab folks' attention. Bariatric surgery is nowhere near the worst decision I ever made. That said, I wish I could go back and tell myself some things before the journey began. There are a lot of things I wish I knew, and a lot of heartache that could've been avoided. There were definitely times when I felt it was the worst decision I ever made, and I want to be able to go back to myself during those times and say, "Hey, man. It'll be ok. You'll get this done. I know that Doctor is a dumbass. In the end, it won't matter."

I would tell myself to make sure to start the actual surgery proceedings early in the calendar year. I definitely recommend this if you have health insurance with a maximum out of pocket amount that rolls over each year. Tell your doctor you want to start doing all the tests, sleep studies, psych exams, and other preparations in January or February if possible. We waited until almost September and, even though we had the sleep studies done, we almost didn't make it. Without insurance, I venture to guess the whole thing would've cost each of us around $30,000. With insurance, it cost both of us $7,000 together. It would've cost us twice that had we both gotten our surgeries done at the beginning of 2018 instead.

Make sure you find a good surgeon. Find one you like, if you can. We got lucky. Our surgeon was excellent, even though the bariatric center she belonged to was an absolute train wreck, and the hospital was a dumpster fire. Given the choice, I would take a good surgeon in a bad office over the opposite any day. The bad office just makes the road to the surgery a pain in the ass.

Don't let your bariatric center, surgical office, doctor's office, or whatever they call themselves be a pain in the ass. Hold them to task. They exist to help you get through the surgery and be healthy, but do not expect them to hold your hand. Do your own research. Know what you need. Know what your insurance company needs. Know what your surgeon needs. Every insurance company, office, and surgeon are different. Just because Amanda and I needed ultrasounds or CT scans doesn't mean you will, and just because we didn't need a colonoscopy doesn't mean you won't. I hope you won't. Ick.

One of my biggest gripes with our bariatric center was that they never gave us a clear picture of the roadmap to our surgery. They gave us a list of tasks, an incomplete one, and told us to get started. They never gave us an order to do the tasks in, expected dates to have them done, or anything like that. Once we were done, they would throw more tasks at us, and then some more, all the way up to the week before our surgery. It was incredibly frustrating. If I were to go back and talk to myself day one, I would at least give myself the order to do things in.

First, get into a nutritionist program. Most insurance companies need at least three months of continuous nutritionist supervision prior to getting surgery, but some need as long as a year or more. Next, get the blood work done. You never know what might show up that needs more tests, and some tests may take a while to schedule or perform. Make sure your family doctor or general practitioner knows what you're doing. Don't expect them to talk or share information with the surgeon or surgeon's office, even though they should. Your GP might have questions or concerns about your blood work that the surgeon doesn't, and it's best to know sooner, rather than later. Avoid surprises.

If it's required, get the sleep study done as soon as possible. Just like the nutritionist, many insurance companies require you to be under the care of a sleep specialist for several months before they will approve the surgery. Most of us overweight folks have sleep apnea, so it's likely that you do if you're contemplating surgery. If you can, avoid having the study done by a hospital or at a hospital, unless you have one you really like. I would recommend getting it done by a private clinic. They tend to have better facilities.

Keep in mind that many of the other procedures are time sensitive, so the results are only good for a limited time. Make sure you have all your pre-existing conditions and other related medical issues signed off on and understood by your surgeon's office before you start doing time sensitive items, like the endoscopy, EKG, x-rays, and psych exams. Schedule those procedures far in advance, but only get them done when just about everything else for the surgery is locked in and ready to go. We were under such a time crunch that we couldn't do that and had to scramble at every turn. Had we started earlier in the year and given ourselves more time, that wouldn't have been such an issue.

Make sure you know where you are in the process at all times and make sure your surgeon's office knows where you are too. I can't count the number of times I talked to someone in our bariatric center and they asked me to verify if I had or had not done something yet. They were either too busy or too disorganized to look it up, and if I told them wrong, they would've just blissfully gone on with planning until they did some actual research, and it was too late to fix. Make them give you a definitive list of tasks, requirements, and expectations. Had I done that, the A1C issue wouldn't have come up for me like it did.

I would've warned myself to lay off the sweets too. If I had done that, the A1C issue wouldn't have come up for me like it did, either.

Even though the road was bumpy, there were several things Amanda and I did right. We found an amazing surgeon to start with. I did a little research on her before we decided to use her and found that she originally came from a major metropolitan area. She had quite a lot of experience, without being old and unwilling to experiment. Not to say that a surgeon from our own part of the country would've been bad, but a surgeon from a larger metropolitan area is probably a safer bet.

We used the buddy system a lot. It was nice to be able to rely on each other to make appointments and yell at the bariatric center employees. When one of us got tired of the stress, the other could take over. We could make appointments for each other, and often together, so that was incredibly helpful. I would suggest you find a sort of surgery buddy if you don't already have one. It's great to have someone to complain to and worry to, should the need arise.

One thing that helped us a great deal was preparing for our liquid diets. We absolutely dreaded the thought of not eating for weeks in a row, so we did a lot of research into protein drinks and other options, such as sugar free popsicles, to break the monotony and help get us the nutrition we needed. We purchased a sample pack of protein powder months before the surgery and spent a week trying every flavor. Once we had a couple flavors we liked, we ordered a big bucket full. The protein powder, along with a couple of ready-made protein drinks we liked from local stores, made the liquid diet bearable if not enjoyable. We still drink many of those drinks to this day.

The last thing I would tell myself is to understand that everyone is different. No matter what you read in this book, or read online, or hear from friends or relatives, your surgery will be different. I get the hiccups, Amanda does not. Amanda had intense abdominal gas pain in the hospital. Mine wasn't as bad, but I had swallowing pain she did not. My dad had the gas pain, and the hiccups, but not the swallowing pain I had. I talked to a girl in one of the post-op classes I attended who could not keep food down, even after almost six weeks. I was eating soft food within two weeks. Most folks say they can't tolerate peanut butter for up to six months after surgery. I've had it almost every day since my third week. It's good protein.

Hitching on to the back of that same wagon, I'll say this: Amanda and I are obviously not following the doctor's orders in regard to diet during our recovery. We also broke quite a few rules leading up to our surgery. I do not recommend doing so. As I've said before, we took our health into our own hands, and you would be doing so too if you decide to go against doctor's orders. We felt that, because everyone is so different, and the doctor's orders are so universal, there was wiggle room for us to cheat a bit. Don't do that. It's bad, and we should feel bad.

After it was all said and done, I don't know that bariatric surgery was really the best, or the worst, decision I ever made. Marrying my wife, graduating college, cancelling DirecTV... all of those rank up there with some of my best decisions. Conversely, things I did in junior high that resulted in my arrest, which are none of your damn business, would rank with some of the worst decisions I've ever made. Bariatric surgery falls in-between those things, but I would definitely put it in the top five. Maybe even top three, though that's a pretty hard sell, considering the options. I suppose if Amanda gets pregnant then I can bump cancelling DirecTV down a notch.

If you're considering it, and I think it's a good chance you are if you're reading this book, then I can do nothing but recommend it. It has changed my life for the better in every way. I don't worship food anymore. As the old cliché goes, I eat to live not live to eat. Even so, I can still eat the things I love, and I still love to eat. Now, I just love to look good doing it, too.

If you or a loved one are having surgery, I wish you the best of health and the best of luck. If you've already had the surgery then congratulations, and I hope everything is going well. If this book helped you, or if you have any questions about what my wife and I went through, please let me know. You can email me any time at edzenisek@gmail.com. I can't promise to respond, but I will try my best.

And, hey, if you see a fat guy from New Mexico eating a big ol' green chile cheeseburger and knocking back a cold one, say hello. That's not me, but he could probably use a friend.

Made in the USA
Columbia, SC
13 April 2018